Sexier Sex

Lessons from

the Brave New Sexual Frontier

REGINA LYNN

SEAL PRE

Sexier Sex
Lessons from the Brave New Sexual Frontier

Copyright © 2008 Regina Lynn

Published by Seal Press
A Member of the Perseus Books Group
1700 Fourth Street
Berkeley, California 94710

Library of Congress Cataloging-in-Publication Data

Lynn, Regina
  Sexier sex: lessons from the brave new sexual frontier / by Regina Lynn.
    p. cm
 ISBN-13: 978-1-58005-231-3
 ISBN-10: 1-58005-231-2
 1. Sex—Miscellanea. 2. Sex—Social aspects. 3. Love. I. Title

HQ23.L94 2008
306.77–dc22

                              2007039419

Cover design by Susan Koski Zucker
Interior design by Tabitha Lahr
Printed in the U.S.A.

To Seth, without whom there would be no book

Contents

ꙮ PART II: FLIRTING ꙮ

ꙮ PART III: SELF-EXPRESSION ꙮ

ℭℓℓ PART IV: JUST LOOKING ℭℓℓ

ℭℓℓ PART V: LOVE ℭℓℓ

PART VI: SEX

PART VII: IDENTITY

ꙮ PART VIII: SAFETY ꙮ

Introduction

Have you ever wanted to dance sexy for a roomful of strangers in a safe environment and see what happened next?

Have you ever wanted to explore sides of your sexual self that you're not quite ready to reveal to your best friend?

Have you ever thought there might be a voyeur . . . a seductress . . . an erotic storyteller . . . a dominatrix . . . a polyamorous, polysexual goddess . . . lurking just beneath your "nice girl" exterior?

Of course you have. And so have thousands of women just like you.

Every day, we are exploring our sexuality in ways that have never before been available to us. And what we're discovering can lead to greater satisfaction and pleasure in our love lives regardless of our relationship status or sexual orientation.

TECHNOLOGY IS A WOMAN'S WORLD

This book is a humorous guide with a serious purpose: helping you expand your sexual horizons in a safe, supportive way. You might choose to try all of the lessons included, or to start with just one. You can skip any that don't appeal to you, do them out of order, modify them to fit your preferences, pleasures, and circumstances.

I provide a wide variety of things to try and to think about. This is by no means an exhaustive list of what you can do with technology and sex. Think of it instead as a starting point to spark your own creative ideas for using your everyday gadgets and gizmos to enhance your relationships.

This book is not about getting yourself into trouble with your partner or giving you excuses to explore sexuality in ways that you know will cause hurt or harm to someone who loves you. Try not to slip into denial about how your actions affect your relationships, particularly if you have children.

This book is also not about fixing anything, either.

My guess is you're probably fine the way you are and you're reading this book because you're curious and want to have a good time. Many women have healed broken hearts, negative self-images, and sexual fears through the kinds of activities outlined in this book. I'm one of them myself.

If you're not in a healthy place to have relationships then your relationships won't be healthy, whether online or off. But you can get to a healthy place—and some of these lessons might help you get there. But keep in mind, I'm no doctor and this is no treatment program.

ISN'T SEX-TECH DANGEROUS?

I've spent the past dozen years experiencing, observing, and analyzing how technology influences romantic relationships, and I have to say, it's not nearly as scary as the mainstream news would have you believe.

If you approach sex-tech with an open mind and a willingness to experiment, you can take these modern tools and add fun, pleasure, and intimacy to your sex life. After all, technology is never going to replace personal relationships, and no one with half a brain wants it to.

Instead we have an opportunity to play in new ways with an age-old game. Anything we don't like, we don't have to do or do again. But those things we do like? How wonderful to have the option!

ABOUT THESE LESSONS

Many of these lessons refer to specific websites, products, and services. These are the ones that I use; they are not the only examples, and they may not be the ones that you like best. The concepts apply across all brands, and in most cases the specific steps will be similar enough that it won't be difficult to adapt them to whichever equivalent you find yourself with.

Technology changes fast, and it's possible that the product's wording or design will have changed between press time and the moment you pick a lesson. Again, let the concepts guide you. Like sex, you can't always predict what is going to happen, so the best thing you can do is relax and embrace the unexpected.

A NOTE ABOUT CATEGORIES AND HEAT METERS

One woman's thrill is another woman's chill—and I'm the last person who wants to yuk your yum. Still, in the interest of putting this book into some sort of organized order, I've gathered the tutorials into categories: Self-Discovery, Flirting, Self-Expression, Just Looking, Love, Sex, Identity, and Safety. Each lesson can be read on its own and independently of all the other lessons, and the thermometer gives you a sense for how "daring" a particular activity is. Here's the legend:

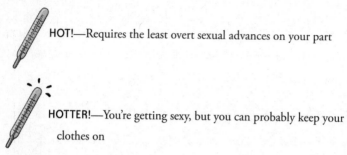

HOT!—Requires the least overt sexual advances on your part

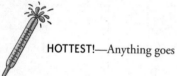

HOTTER!—You're getting sexy, but you can probably keep your clothes on

HOTTEST!—Anything goes

So dive on in. Check it out. Get experimental. And have some fun while you're at it.

Part I:

Self - Discovery

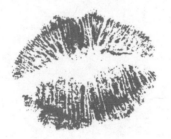

Eliza Doolittle would not have needed 'enry 'iggins as the catalyst for finding herself had she been able to go online.

Time just moves faster in cyberspace. We learn so much about ourselves in such a short time when we're online. You might discover you have an eye for fetish photography, or that playing a pin-up girl online has made you more confident offline. If you've always felt like something was missing, but you're not sure what, you can find out what it is by venturing into places online that you couldn't set foot in offline (at least not yet).

Some of us find ourselves counseling others online about their relationships and realize we actually do know what our next move should be in our own lives. Others find that getting sexy with other regular people opens our eyes to the potential of the nice guy or gal next door whose looks didn't blow us away but who has that . . . gleam . . . in the eye.

You may have noticed that people make snide comments and uncomfortable jokes about the role of the Internet in masturbation—but we women know that if we don't know how to give ourselves pleasure, we can't expect anyone else to know how either. The discomfort around online play stems from a deeply rooted and unfortunate discomfort with masturbation itself, not from an informed perspective on what the technology can do for us.

This section contains lessons that apply specifically to learning more about yourself and your sexuality.

How to Buy Lingerie for Your Body Type

 HOT!

It seems like lingerie is designed for women who are 5' 6", wear a 34C bra, size 5 panties, and size 7 shoes—unless you are that woman and still have fit problems, in which case, I guess it's designed for our avatars rather than our bodies.

And when lingerie doesn't fit, we blame ourselves for being too short or tall, too fat or thin, too busty or too flat, too long in the torso or too thick in the calf.

Shopping for lingerie online eliminates a lot of the hassles. It might seem counterintuitive, as with fit troubles you want to be able to try it on. But when you shop online, you can quickly narrow your options to just the negligee that is likely to fit. You can try it on in your own bedroom with your own lighting and your own mirror, and if you hate it, send it back. (Yes, this can cost money, but you won't begrudge it after you find something that makes you feel like a million bucks.)

And most likely, if you put the effort into the search, you won't hate it.

★ Don't rely on size chart measurements. Email or call the site with your measurements and notes about your proportions, how other brands and sizes fit you, and what you're looking for.

INTIMATE SHOPPING

Figleaves.com
Cups from A to JJ, bands from 28 to 54. Need I say more?

StormyLeather.com
Leather clothing (and toys), both ready to wear and couture.

Trashy.com
Beverly Hills institution, known for custom garments and costumes.

HipsandCurves.com
Lingerie that celebrates full, voluptuous curves.

Bravissimo.com
Great selection of bras in D cup and up, plus clothing designed to fit and flatter busty figures.

★ Shop internationally. You pay a bit more in shipping, but it's worth it if you get the right fit.

★ Stockings, stretchy chemises, and collars fit just about everyone. It doesn't matter if the stockings won't stay up if you're just wearing them on nights in.

★ More coverage can be as sexy as less, especially in sheer fabrics. Lingerie is less about skin as it is about mystery. Especially as we get older.

★ Forget the size noted on the label and look only for fit. I have lingerie that ranges from size M to size 2X, and it all fits me exactly the same.

★ If your proportions are impossible to fit off the rack, investigate custom services. There is nothing wrong with your body—only with the narrow range of fits available.

★ Corsets look fantastic on all body shapes, but must be custom-made to look perfect.

How to Improve Your
Body Image in Five Easy Steps

 HOT!

It might seem odd to turn to the Internet to boost your body image, as the general idea is that when we go online, we leave our bodies behind. Yet what better way to shed body worries than to engage with others without your body? Remember how intelligent, funny, and downright sexy you are when you're not worrying about your waistband?

Playing on the Internet can help you become more comfortable in your own skin long after you log off. That same wit and sensuality you radiate online still lives within you the rest of the time; the more you practice letting it out, the more natural it becomes. (And then you have to be careful not to let loose at inappropriate times, like job interviews!)

Body confidence is sexy and infuses every dimension of our lives, not just sex.

★ Set up your webcam and practice posing until you find a few positions and angles that please you. This is like those body-image exercises performed in front of a mirror, except the tiny frame and the semi-grainy quality of the

> *Sex appeal is 50 percent what you've got and 50 percent what people think you've got.*
>
> —Sophia Loren

picture create an entirely different experience, as does the knowledge that once you do start seeing your body in terms of the beauty of its lights and shadows, you can share it with other people with a few clicks. (See "How to Look Great on Webcam," page 111)

★ Unless all porn truly offends you, surf amateur porn to see the wide range of bodies engaged in sex. Sex often looks ridiculous, but bodies in lusty pursuits are also rather beautiful, especially when you can see the erotic or emotional connection among the participants.

★ Flirt shamelessly in text and dazzle others with your inventiveness and wickedness. The more time you spend feeling alluring and sexy, the more you realize that you *are* alluring and sexy. And when you figure that out, it's natural to bring that confidence into all aspects of your life.

★ Learn to make love to your cell phone camera—purse your lips, take interesting close-ups of your face or a lock of hair, get a fun picture of your freshly pedicured toes. I always hold my phone above and slightly to the side of my face to emphasize my eyes and cheekbones. So often, we focus so closely on what we dislike about our bodies that we forget we have assets too.

★ If you're single or if your partner is cool with it, have cybersex. All those endorphins and hours of sexual attention awaken the earthy, sensual side and prove that sexuality is just as much a mind thing as a body thing—and the more you exercise your sexy brain, the more you notice your sexy body.

How to Keep Your
Sense of Humor

 HOT!

If you know anything about technology, you know that it
is a capricious, mischievous beast. And if you know anything about sex, you
know that it too can be ridiculous, poignant, and hilarious by turns. Combining
the two sometimes feels like the biggest joke on earth.

It's enough to make you want to cry.

You visit a chat room once or twice "just to see" and soon find yourself
deeply involved in a romantic triangle more dramatic than a historical romance.
Your heart swings up and down each time you log in, your Internet connection
seems to know exactly when to go on the fritz, and your patience is tested to the
limit by the vagaries of time zones, work schedules, family life, and idiots who
enter the chat room solely for the purpose of annoying you.

The only way to reap the benefits of online exploration is to accept technical
and other difficulties as part of the experience. An amusing part, if you can. It's
easy for outsiders to dismiss online activity as fantasy—I refer to it that way
myself sometimes, for convenience. But it's no utopia: This "fantasy" world has
its full share of tricksters and trolls.

A sense of humor is your best defense against all of it, including criticisms
and teasing from your friends when they find you've been moonlighting as
SexyPaloma. These tips will help you keep your perspective.

WHEN TECH GOES BAD

★ Internet connections seem to know just when you've started interacting in a romantic or erotic way, particularly if it's a wireless signal. Reconnect as quickly as you can, dismiss it with a joke (". . . and that, my liege, is how we know the Earth to be banana-shaped" or "Did anybody get the plates of the Mack truck that just hit me?"), and get back into the conversation. Dwelling on the frustration just sours the conversation for everyone involved.

★ Cell phones do the same thing. You'll be having a perfectly fine conversation, flirting like a pro, and then it's time to convey the most important information. Maybe a time and place to meet, or an email address to send pictures to—and suddenly, you might as well be on Mars. All you can do is laugh and repeat yourself. And follow up with a text message, which often gets through when voice gets garbled.

★ If one technology lets you down, try another. Email sometimes works when instant messaging doesn't. If Skype goes down, try Yahoo or MSN audio chat. If you play in a 3D world and you're traveling and stuck on dialup, go retro with a text-only chat room, or even—gasp—have the person call your motel phone.

★ When you do finally get connected, try not to spend a lot of time cursing the tech or dwelling on the frustration. Not only does that waste precious minutes, it seems to inspire the technology to give you even more troubles.

WHEN PEOPLE FORGET TO CHILL

★ Most of the time, the best defense against hecklers is simply to ignore them. (Most community tools have a Block or Ignore button for that very purpose.) But ignoring them in public doesn't mean you aren't annoyed, hurt, or angry inside. In that case, you've got to step back and take a breath. If you can keep your conversation light and funny, other people in the community will follow your lead and engage with you and ignore the jerks too. Once the jerks discover they can't control the room, they generally leave.

★ Online romance gets very dramatic very quickly. That's part of its appeal— and part of why it looks so ridiculous to those on the outside. If you can manage to laugh at yourself from time to time, your pairings will be healthier and more manageable.

★ It seems to be an online tradition to snark at people when they express themselves. No matter how you express yourself, blogging, chatting, pictures, whatever, someone is going to say something nasty. But you know what? Every time someone posts a comment, it boosts your traffic count. And if you ever want to sell advertising or promote your work, traffic is one of the most important things you can show. Rather than snark back or get in flame wars in your comments, fend it off with a joke if you can think of a good one, or simply ignore it. Whatever you do, don't take it personally—people who go online specifically to tear other people down are not worth your time or energy.

How to Justify the Expense of Luxury Sex Toys, and Why

 HOT!

In the past couple of years, high-end sex toys have taken the adult novelty market by storm. With expensive materials, quality manufacturing, and beautiful aesthetics in both design and packaging, these swanky products put the $20 plastic battery vibes to shame.

And yet even women who think nothing of spending $200 or more on a pair of boots hesitate at the price tags of the most elegant adult products. For some reason, we don't feel that our pleasure is important enough to invest serious cash in, especially if we're in a relationship and feel guilty about spending money on sexual delights we intend to use mostly by ourselves. (Although really, anything you can use with yourself, you can use with your partner.)

And yet more and more, we're accepting that sex toys are just another household appliance. You wouldn't skimp on a washing machine or a blender, now would you? Or how about that flat panel TV?

If you're still not sure, consider this:

★ Orgasms relieve stress, increase circulation, improve your skin, and make you feel closer to your lover.

★ The more sex you have, the more sex you want. (Use it or lose it!)

★ Giving your body pleasure teaches you how to give and accept even more pleasure with a lover.

★ Sexual pleasure boosts your mood, long after the lovemaking is over.

★ High-end sex toys last longer and feel better than their cheaper cousins.

★ Luxury toys are likely to come with a warranty and a beautiful box or pouch for storage.

★ A toy that is beautiful to look at inspires you to want to use it, and doesn't break the mood when you bring it into partner play.

★ Stores that carry these more expensive lines are staffed with sex educators who can help you find toys that suit your desires so you don't have to worry about spending $100 or more on a product you're not going to like.

★ Makers of elegant toys use the best-quality materials and designs. You won't encounter sharp seams, strong chemical smells, or peeling coatings in this product range.

★ A quality device lasts years longer than the cheap ones. You're not wasting money, you're investing in something that will give you pleasure for a long time.

How to Turn Your MP3 Player into a Personal Pleasure Device

HOTTER!

Remember the joy of the mix tape, crafted especially for you by that special someone? Here's a variation on that theme for adults only. There are vibrators that pulse, rev, and throb to the beat of audio sources, ranging from a music playlist to your lover's voice right there in bed.

For a group experience, try plugging one into your computer headphone jack and meeting up in a chat room or a virtual world where you can all groove to the same audio stream.

These toys are available at most reputable adult retailers, or you can Google them to find the best deals.

IBUZZ TWO

Comes with two small vibrators to put inside a bunny-shaped sleeve for her and a cock ring for him—and all the necessary connecting cables, including a headphone splitter so you can both listen to the same music while you wear your toys.

OHMIBOD

A slim, insertable vibrator in colors to complement the iPod and iPhone, although any device with a headphone jack will drive it. Comes in a pretty zippered pouch for tucking discreetly into your purse and has "penis sleeve" accessories to create different textures and looks apart from the basic cylinder. Visit Club Vibe at www.ohmibod.com for a playlist exchange among OhMiBod users and special playlists created by professional DJs, all mixed specifically for their vibratory delights.

TALK2ME

This beautifully sculpted dual-purpose toy splits the incoming audio into two streams; the vibrating shaft responds to the bass, while the tickler responds to the treble. You can hook it up to a headphone jack or set its wireless receiver in front of any source of sound—your lips, your stereo, your motorcycle—and get your groove on.

How to Research Your Sexual Health

 HOT!

The great thing about the Internet is that it has brought so much health information to your fingertips.

The bad thing about the Internet is that it has brought so much health information to your fingertips.

Face it: How often do you go online to check out a symptom, only to realize you are one hangnail away from lifelong disability or even . . . death?

Yet when it comes to sexual health, the Internet is a woman's best friend. While I don't believe we should be embarrassed to discuss anything with our doctors, including sex, I do know that not all of us have open-minded healthcare professionals. Nor do we always have the opportunity to change practitioners the moment one reveals prejudices around our sexual lifestyles, practices, or behaviors.

The first thing a modern woman does when she finds a suspicious lump, red mark, or discharge is go online for reassurance that it's just an ingrown hair or a yeast infection. Unfortunately, that's not always the case. And as my mom says, not knowing doesn't make something not true.

It's normal to arm yourself with information—and even make yourself paranoid—before you head to the doctor. Yet the Internet being what it is, how do you know you're looking at reliable information?

You can't really. Even the Centers for Disease Control and Prevention has been rumored to fudge sexual health information due to political pressure to promote abstinence and prevent abortions.

The best strategy is to visit a variety of resources and pull together a good picture of what the literature says. I'm a big fan of forums, because you can find out how other people deal with sexual health issues. This is the epitome of women using the web to better their lives, as they share stories and solutions and realize that they are not alone in any of their fears or concerns. Women can also help each other formulate questions to take to appointments with health care professionals and compare notes afterwards. Then, when you go to your appointment, you're armed with the terminology and the questions to ask.

Here are some reliable places to start.

WEBMD.COM

My go-to site for all things health-related, sexual and otherwise. I have found the user forums there particularly helpful, because you can talk with real people who have the same conditions and face the same challenges when communicating with partners, family members, and health professionals.

SEXUALITY.ABOUT.COM

Sex educator Cory Silverberg maintains an excellent repository of sexual health information. He is particularly helpful if you are looking for information about how to enjoy a healthy sex life despite challenges like disability, injury, or pain.

SCARLETEEN.COM

Sexual health information for teenagers that's also useful for grown-up women who haven't been single in a long time. If the last time you bought a condom, you sought out one with nonoxynol-9, or if the worst STD you could get in your wilder days was herpes, don't be embarrassed to start here.

APHRODITEWOMENSHEALTH.COM/FORUMS

These are lively message boards where you can talk to other women about sexual concerns and conditions. Based in Australia, the all-woman team behind Aphrodite Women's Health is focused on providing information and forums —and since they are web publishers and community facilitators, not health professionals, they don't push their medical perspectives at you.

NURTUREYOURNATURE.ORG

A joint effort of the Association of Reproductive Health Professionals (ARHP) and the National Women's Health Resource Center (NWHRC) to bring female sexual health and wellness into the public eye.

GOASKALICE.COM

Another resource aimed at young adults; it also contains a wealth of information for us older folk.

How to Discover (and Free) Your Erotic Imagination

HOTTER!

Many of the lessons in the book encourage you to exercise your erotic imagination. But what if you don't feel very imaginative? What if you can't picture being turned on by an imaginary experience? What if it's been so long since you let your desires into the light, you don't even remember what they are?

You have two choices. You can decide imagination is not for you and skip this lesson in favor of more practical topics. Or you can coax your mind to remember its role as the most important sex organ, and enrich your love life, whatever it happens to be.

One way to lure your fantasy life out of its cave is to go online and talk sex with other people. If the boundaries of your relationship prevent that, you might read an erotica message board or listen to erotic podcasts to engage your imagination.

PERMISSION

Give yourself permission to spend time and effort imagining sex—and enjoying it (see "How to Give Yourself Permission" on page 27 for more.). (If you need someone else's permission, you have mine.) Anything that turns you on is fair game, even if you think your mom, your church, or even your partner would think it taboo. Thoughts are not deeds, and while we all need to try to keep our deeds from causing harm, we're just talking about imagination here. Chances are your fantasies harm no one.

START WITH A THEME

If you've been stressed and tired for a long, long time, it's hard to shift gears and let your mind play. Start with a cliché: There's a reason certain themes appear again and again in sexual fantasy. Think beaches, waterfalls, palaces, dungeons, mountains. Think strangers, princes, movie stars, evil yet strangely compelling spacefaring pirates. Is it a rescue, a seduction, a kidnapping? All of these and more are being played out online in chat rooms, audio chat, and virtual worlds, with personal embellishments and touches that make each fantasy new again for the lovers.

ACCEPT FEELING SILLY

If you worry that you are being silly or dramatic, so what? It's sex. It's fantasy. It's going to be dramatic, otherwise there's no story. If you let your anxieties go and flow with the fantasy you are building, either through reading and writing stories or through interacting with other people, your body gets a chance to relax into the mood.

SEEK RICH ENVIRONMENTS

Virtual worlds like Second Life, Jewel of Indra, and Red Light Center put you right there in the setting of your fantasy. You don't have to picture the waterfall from scratch, because someone has already built it. If you don't like it, you can build one of your own.

Virtual worlds can be intimidating at first, especially if you've never played video games and are not familiar with concepts like "inventory," "avatars," "sim," and the like. The best way to get started is to sign up and follow the directions for creating a basic avatar—your digital self—and then enter the world. Upon entry, you will be in a "welcome" or "orientation" area, and you will see a box where you can type a message and introduce yourself to the people around you. Something like "Hi, I'm Aphrodite! This is my first time here, so I'm trying to figure everything out" is often answered by offers to help you, show you around and teach you the best ways to use the controls. (See "How to Get Started in Virtual Worlds" on page 143 for more.)

INTERACT

If you're single or in a relationship that permits outside exploration, get into an adult community online and start talking. Nothing frees the erotic imagination more than sharing a sexual experience with someone, building the story as you go, responding to each other's contributions and—perhaps—even including an orgasm or two of your own.

How to Give
Yourself Permission

 HOT!

"You're the perfect person to grant permission," my friend tells me, "for the exact reason that you don't get why people ask for it."

It's true. I can't remember the last time I asked permission for anything but the obvious, like borrowing someone's power drill or eating the last strawberry or putting my finger—well, you get the idea.

Even though I'm not an advice columnist, I get a lot of email asking for advice. What I've found is that most of the time, the writers already know what they want to do. They just need someone to tell them it's okay to do it.

Permission ultimately has to come from within. But sometimes it's hard to give ourselves permission until someone else—externally—grants it to us as well.

I see this especially with adults who were molested as children, or who survived rape or abusive sexual relationships, or who live with repression and guilt and fear. They often worry greatly that their own sexual desires are somehow perverted or degrading or evil. They want external guidelines to follow before they can develop the confidence to create an internal framework of what they consent to sexually and what they don't.

It doesn't help that the media constantly reinforces the idea that combining sex and tech in any way automatically makes you a pervert, a loser, or somehow abnormal.

And yet, what's great about sex-tech is that it is fostering a more sexually accepting society in which we can talk about this stuff without feeling unsafe or embarrassed. (If you don't think things are changing radically and globally, just look at the panic about sex in the extreme conservative political agenda, here and abroad.)

We're realizing that we're not alone in our desires or lack thereof; even if we feel damaged or abnormal, we realize that many others do too, and we can work through it together. Through the ever-growing online conversation, more of us will find our own comfort level with what is and isn't okay with us sexually—as well as the skill to communicate that comfort level to our partners, both online and off.

The Internet is made for exploration, so explore! In a fantasy space, you can log off at any time if things get too uncomfortable. Therefore, it's not so hard to speak up if your boundaries are being pushed and to ask people to back off when you need them to, because if they continue to press you can simply disappear and find a more welcoming community elsewhere.

Don't be afraid of your sexuality. Let sex-tech open doors for you; you can always close them again if you find out one thing or another is not for you. Once you grant yourself permission to feel good, to explore fantasies and desires in the safety of virtual space, don't be surprised if you grant yourself that same permission in the rest of your sex life.

Feels good, doesn't it?

How to Store
Your Sex Toys

HOT!

Where do you keep your little buddies? In a drawer? A
shoebox? In the dishwasher?

Obviously your toys don't care where you put them as long as they are
protected from dust, direct sunlight, and pets. But storing your toys in an
attractive manner is one way to show yourself and your lovers the importance of
sex and pleasure. It reminds you that you have no reason to be ashamed—and
in fact, every reason to be proud—of your collection and your determination to
make sexuality a priority in your life.

Luxury toys tend to come in lovely packaging, like the velvet-lined locking
chests from Elemental Pleasures and the pink satin nests from nJoy Toys.
Unfortunately, many standard toys for sale are still packaged in pornographic
plastic clamshells you need industrial strength scissors to open.

★ For Your Nymphomation makes cases in a variety of sizes, from condom-
size to toy chest. Each is lockable and features glow-in-the-dark zipper pulls,
faux leather textures, and a variety of colors and designs.

> "A lockable storage case not only protects your privacy (from in-laws, kids, and housekeepers) but also protects your toys (from dust and damage). Why would you spend a lot of money on quality toys and then not store and protect them so they last a long time? Toys are an investment in your sexual happiness. Women generally like to have cases for everything—makeup, sunglasses, cell phone, iPod, laptop, etc., so why not have a case for condoms and adult toys as well? An organized sex life will help with organizing your whole life, and properly protected condoms will properly protect you. Our cases are also loved by men (for hiding porn magazines and DVDs), as well as by the BDSM crowd, for storing their floggers, whips, canes, riding crops, suspension bars, and other equipment and toys."
>
> —Vera Worthington, designer and founder, For Your Nymphomation

★ Hide Your Vibe pillows are the adult version of the stuffed animals with the zippered pouches for your pajamas and toothbrush. Nestle your toys inside, then toss 'em on the bed or sofa, and No One Would Ever Suspect—until they wrap their arms around it to take a nap, that is. You can find them at Amazon.com and several online adult retailers.

★ Kitchen containers (Tupperware, Rubbermaid), plastic shoeboxes, and hat boxes lined with pretty fabrics are inexpensive ways to organize a toy collection, although you'll need to improvise some locks if that's important to you. In fact, you can probably find a number of nice storage options at places like The Container Store.

★ Wouldn't it be fun to explain to a custom closets designer that you want a portion of the unit devoted to your "intimacy collection"?

★ You can keep condoms safe in your purse in a makeup case or a special condom container made of padded cloth or aluminum. A case protects them against punctures, spills, and other wear 'n' tear. It's also a good idea to keep a small LED light in the bag to help you find the condoms in a hurry.

★ Jewelry boxes also make discreet by-the-bed storage for small toys like vibrating rings and butt plugs, and for condoms and dental dams too.

★ Devine Toys makes a variety of locking toy boxes and travel cases, along with a "French envelope" that protects two condoms at a time and the cuter-than-kittens "Condom Cube" that stores a full dozen and even comes in quilted pink *with hearts*. Precious!

How to Furnish
Your Sex Room

 HOT!

We're often told to leave the computer and the TV out of the bedroom and use the bed only for sleeping and sex (and maybe reading, if the relationship counselor is being generous).

I'd rather focus on what we *can* do, rather than what we can't, to make the bedroom (or den, or kitchen—or every room in the house, if you're ambitious) more conducive to lovemaking.

Because this is not an interior decorating book—and believe me, I'm the last person who should be advising anyone on design—I'm going to leave that to you to research elsewhere. But I can help you with a few additional touches for lovers—some overt, and some so subtle that your lover might not even notice.

★ If your bed doesn't have posts, rails, or another easy-to-tie-something-to-it frame design, invest in a personal restraint system from Sportsheet. The bottom sheet fastens to the mattress, and the restraints, wedges, pillows, and props attach to the sheet. Sex shops also sell long straps that go all the way under the mattress and come up on each side for bondage play.

★ Liberator makes cushion props for lovers that blend into other pillows and bedding. The products are made from special materials (developed for use by the space program!) intended to support your body and make certain positions possible without sliding around, squashing down, or otherwise letting you down at the wrong time. If the prices make you gasp with shock rather than arousal, Love Pegasus makes some cheaper alternatives. And if you happen to be in Australia or the UK, check out the Loving Angles modular furniture—they will send you swatches so you can coordinate the colors just right.

★ If you can, keep supplies handy from anywhere on the bed—whatever "supplies" means to you. You don't want to have to travel across a king-size bed to reach the lube! See "How to Store Your Toys" on page 29 for ideas of how you can store sex supplies attractively and discreetly while also placing them within reach.

★ Some people prefer a mirror to face them; others prefer a more oblique angle, so you can look if you want; and some don't want a mirror in the bedroom at all. If you have mirrored closet doors and can't stand the thought of seeing your reflections, invest in blindfolds.

★ Add a chair that's firm enough to support one or both of your bodies in a variety of positions. For oral sex, one can sit while the other kneels. Or one can be bent over the arm, seat, or back while the other penetrates from behind. A wide chair fosters cuddling; a narrow chair works well for straddling the seated partner.

THINGS TO STASH IN SUPPLY CACHES:

★ lube

★ condoms and other safer sex items

★ small toys

★ blindfold

★ a feather

★ honey dust

★ nipple clamps

★ vibrating cock ring

★ washcloth or hand towel or wet napkins

★ breath mints

★ porn

★ cell phone (for those important phone sex dates when one of you is out of town)

★ Or you can skip the regular "reading chair" look and go straight for the real thing. The Tantra Chair has a sensual S curve, comes in two wood finishes and several fabrics, and offers support for all kinds of sensual positions. The Love Rocker looks like exercise equipment, supporting one partner with a series of springs. Users claim it is surprisingly comfortable.

How to Boost Your Libido

HOTTER!

The hamster wheel of modern life diminishes our sex drives every bit as much as illness, chronic pain, or hormonal fluctuations. We don't always have time to eat right, exercise, and get enough sleep—even though we know all of those things improve our sex lives. Many of us feel like we're barely holding up under the combination of work, kids, and chores. Add one or more medications, alcohol use, depression, anxiety, body image issues—sometimes it's a wonder we have sex drives at all.

But don't get too anxious about it. Libido does ebb and flow, and if you get too worried, your anxiety can hinder your sexual response. Talk to your doctor, talk to your partner, talk to your best friend, talk to others online who struggle with the same issues—and be gentle with yourself.

While I'm not thrilled to see the drug companies invent a new disorder—"female sexual dysfunction"—I am glad that female sexual pleasure is finally becoming a priority in our society. And if that's a side effect of the new crop of erection drugs, so be it.

Libido is not just an issue for older women. In my twenties, I took a daily low dose of testosterone for about a year, trying to restore a libido that had succumbed to the weight of my depression. It took a few months to adjust the dose, and it actually did work. When I pulled myself out of the depression (and I'd venture to say that having more sex helped that!), I stopped taking the testosterone. I worried that my libido would plummet, but it didn't, and I was pleased that I had talked to my gynecologist about what, up until then, I had been too embarrassed to mention. (My, how things have changed. . . .)

It's nice that we have some options for those times when our libidos shoot through the basement and we admit to ourselves we'd rather nap or read than even think about touching ourselves or a partner. However, our minds know that sex is important, even when our bodies seem to have forgotten.

I am not a doctor or a health practitioner, and I'm sensitive to side effects to boot, so please don't interpret this lesson as medical advice by any stretch of the imagination. I'm also wary of the topical agents that increase blood flow to the genitals, as that seems like a recipe for intimate irritation, and patches annoy my skin; my body is more comfortable with prescription-based helpers like testosterone pills. But the following will give you an idea of what's out there so you can feel better informed when you talk to your doc about what might work best for your particular body and situation.

PRESCRIPTION

Testosterone can be delivered by a daily pill or skin patch. I used the pills and kept them next to my birth control pills so I wouldn't forget to take them.

OVER THE COUNTER

There are several topical gels and creams that encourage blood flow to the genitals. The active ingredient is usually L-arginine or niacin, both of which cause a warming, sensitizing sensation that can be too much for some women. Be careful when trying these, and have a cool washcloth or a wipe handy in case you need to take it off in a hurry. Also, check the labels to make sure the brand you're trying is condom-safe, if necessary.

AROMATHERAPY

The Scentuelle patch is a "nontransdermal" stick-on that releases subtle, sexy scent molecules through nanotechnology. I'm no chemist, but I can say this: Committing to wearing it for a few weeks makes you more aware of yourself as a sensual being, and people respond to that in very interesting ways. You wear it and take frequent whiffs throughout the day and make your partner a very happy camper throughout the night. (Or vice versa. It's not confined to the clock.)

How to Build a Sex-Tech Collection Your Friends Will Envy

HOTTER!

When shopping for toys, it's always good to talk with a staffer at a sex-positive boutique that has an extensive education program, as they can help guide you to products that fit your preferences.

However.

If you're already pretty sure that you've got everything you need and are now cruising for something you want, here are some of my favorites.

✔ **BEST ORAL SEX SIMULATOR**

Je Joue

✔ **BEST TOTALLY SILENT CYBERSEX CHAIR**

Monkey Rocker

✔ **BEST FIRST TOY FOR COUPLES**

Vibrating cock ring

✔ **BEST ACCESSORY THAT DOUBLES AS A READING PILLOW**
Liberator wedge

✔ **BEST DILDOS FOR THE LIVING ROOM DISPLAY SHELF**
Atraw Ceramics

✔ **BEST EVERYDAY WORKHORSE**
Eroscillator

✔ **BEST SHOWER-FRIENDLY TOY**
Elemental Pleasures

✔ **BEST ECONOMY MODEL VIBE THAT STILL LOOKS LOVELY**
Natural Contours

✔ **BEST TOY THAT DOUBLES AS A HAT RACK**
Fantasy Glide

✔ **BEST BLOW JOB ACCESSORY**
Nexus Glide

✔ **BEST QUICKIE**
Hitachi Magic Wand with G-Spot Accessory

✔ **BEST WAY TO SURPRISE THE PERSON EMPTYING THE DISHWASHER**

nJoy stainless steel butt plugs

✔ **BEST TOY THAT HIDES IN PLAIN SIGHT**

I Rub My Ducky rubber ducky vibrator

How to Use Your
Cell Phone as a Sex Toy

HOTTEST!

What woman hasn't set her phone to vibrate mode and then thought . . . hmmm?

If you have an older phone, you might be able to download the Purring Kitty software at Vibelet.com for less than the price of a latte. This software lets you start the vibration—which will continue until you stop it, or until your battery dies, whichever comes first. Some phones pulse, and some phones keep a steady buzz. Make sure your phone is on the list of compatibles before you buy, however, because there are no refunds.

Another option is the Blissbox Vibe, which has a similar effect and works on Nokia phones.

If the vibration software isn't available to you, go to homemade-sex-toys .com/cellphone for a few crafty tricks to hack your mobile and get it to ring your bell. For example, try setting an alarm for several successive minutes and using the vibrate mode for the alert. Or get a friend to call you several times in a row until you call him back, in a dreamy postorgasm haze, and thank him profusely.

"As a 45-year-old who had to teach most of her friends what texting was and how to do it, I'm surprised to find that my 50-year-old manfriend loves to have text-sex. It's a fun secret between us."

—S.

But vibration is not the only way your mobile can become an instrument of pleasure. For one thing, it has a camera for a reason. It might even have video. What's stopping you from recording a daily video message and sending it to your lover's email?

It doesn't have to be X-rated to be erotic. If you don't quite trust that your new flame won't post it to MySpace, use objects with suggestive shapes to create sensual imagery without your face or other body parts in the frame. The last eight inches of a broom handle backlit behind a sheet makes an interesting picture—and you can step behind that sheet yourself to get naughty without being too exposed.

If video is too much, a "good morning" picture, sent at 9:00 AM on the dot every workday, can be a sweet routine for both of you. Especially if you vary the pictures to match your mood. All it takes is one or two "special" shots to keep a person wondering what goodies he might get today.

Get two headsets so you can talk hands-free—one to keep in the car for commuting conversations, and the other to keep in your purse for naughty talk any time, any place. Imagine having an erotic exchange entirely in code, so those people walking by have no idea what you're really thinking about on your lunchtime walk.

Yes, it's rude to impose your phone conversation on others in many venues, like restaurants and trains. But if you're striding down the sidewalk, you're hardly interfering with someone else's space, so go for it. Just make sure you remember to speak in your secret language—there's nothing like an ill-timed "cock" or "pussy" to attract unwanted attention.

How to Stay Sex-Savvy
and Not Be Fooled by Internet
"Experts" Who Aren't

HOTTER!

One of the greatest roles the Internet plays in modern sexuality is that it makes sex information available to everyone who can get online. The flip side: Not all of that information is reliable. And to paraphrase Dr. Charlie Glickman, director of education at Good Vibrations, not having the right information about sex can land you in the emergency room.

It's also not always easy to find all the sex information you need in one place. Sex encompasses so many niches: medical, biological, emotional, social.

And the Internet makes it so easy for people to build up reputations as "experts," even thought they really aren't. (That's one reason I always remind people who email me that I'm a "woman in the field," not a licensed counselor!)

These are some of the questions I ask when I evaluate a new source.

★ Is the sex expert certified by the American Association of Sexuality Educators, Counselors and Therapists (AASECT)?

★ Do bloggers I respect link to this person or site often?

★ Does the information have a particular political bias or agenda? For me, it's okay if it does, but it needs to be up front about it.

★ How old is the expert? I do not mean to be ageist, but I respect experience. I'm more likely to trust a forty-three-year-old relationship writer than a college sex columnist.

★ Where has this person been published?

★ Where does this person teach? A person who has taught at Good Vibrations U, Babeland, or the Center for Sex and Culture is likely to be someone who knows their stuff.

★ Who is the audience for this source? Does the site reach that audience? If a site is trying to act like it's a professional journal but its content and design are all pop culture, I stay away.

★ How does this person behave toward contrary opinion and detractors of their viewpoint? How professional is this person in communication style?

★ Does this source cite specific, credible studies to support his or her views?

How to Find
Sex Therapy Online

HOTTER!

Imagine a future where sex therapy, sex educators, and sex partners are available to you at any time of day, in your own house, ready to help you with whatever you need at the moment.

Oh, hey. That would be . . . right now.

If connecting online feels natural and right to you, the Internet is a natural place to seek therapy. You're already accustomed to peer support through online interaction; why wouldn't you reach for a professional in the same way?

Online therapy is particularly suited to sex and relationship work, especially if you need a layer of anonymity you can't get by going through your insurance company or driving to an office. You can seek matches based on compatibility rather than proximity.

But you also have to commit to doing the work if you want to get anything out of it. That means copping to your true feelings, even if that's not how you want to present yourself. By its very nature, e-therapy forces us to acknowledge and express our emotions honestly in order to work.

"E-therapy teaches clients to be aware of what's coming out of their mouths, what they're feeling and thinking, their wholeness and whole bodies. It's an exciting and empowering thing that we haven't done in the past (in person) the way we can with text. Text is really powerful."

—Susan Mankita, LCSW, social work consultant and educator in Miami, who has been training mental health professionals about online practice since 1995.

Without a counselor in the room, there is no audience to perform for. Just you, your honesty, and a diary that writes back.

In person, you can hope the therapist tunes in to your body language, providing a bridge between feeling an emotion and expressing it. In text, you not only have to pay attention to your emotions, you have to recognize them and express them yourself.

A WORD ABOUT PRIVACY

While online counseling offers a lot of personal privacy, make sure you take precautions about your digital privacy as well. Some virtual offices have encryption tools for all of your correspondence, but some just use regular email. Make sure you create a separate account with a password no one would ever guess. If you're concerned about family members stumbling upon your work, create a separate email account with a password they would never guess, and don't forget to clear your browser cache after each use.

WHERE TO FIND AN E-THERAPIST

International Society for Mental Health Online

www.Ismho.org

Professional organization setting standards for quality, effective e-therapy

eTherapistsOnline

www.etherapistsonline.com

A network of counselors offering live chat, email, and phone sessions

Online Clinics

www.onlineclinics.com

A directory of e-therapists who use Online Clinics for secure private "web offices"

PsychCentral

http://psychcentral.org

A complete mental health resource, with support groups and professional therapists

Relationship Help Online

www.relationshiphelponline.com.au

A service offered by non-profit organization Relationships Australia to extend counseling services to people who can't make it to appointments in person or who prefer the convenience and anonymity of online therapy.

Women aren't as instantly good at this as you might think. We're good at tuning into emotion, particularly emotion in other people, but we're also good at fooling ourselves or trying to present ourselves as more "pulled together" than we really feel.

Just as online flirting and cybersex can improve our sex lives, practicing this emotional work in text is a great way to learn how to be more communicative and honest about our feelings overall. And that leads to being more relaxed and more adult in our relationships.

How to Shop for Sex Toys from the Comfort of Your Own Home

HOTTER!

It sounds obvious. Go to Amazon.com or Drugstore.com and order a new vibrator. It's no more difficult—and no more exciting—than ordering light bulbs.

But what if you want something more? Maybe you have special requirements, like a silent vibrator your roommates or kids won't hear from the next room. Maybe you're ready for a luxury device, and you need a better idea of what you'll get for your $150. Or maybe you are dealing with an injury or a physical limitation that makes the standard shapes and switches difficult to manage.

What you want is a shop with professional sex educators who can give you information about sex—not just about the product. All of the stores listed in this lesson offer educational features, tutorials, recommendations, and other useful stuff for how a particular toy can fit into your life. If you don't find your answers on the sites, give them a call or drop them a line, and they will be happy to guide you.

You can also read the articles and watch the tutorials alone or with your partner—they are great ice breakers and can offer you a helping hand for starting a conversation that shouldn't be difficult but for some reason often is.

For example, if you say "I love feeling you inside me, and I would like us to try one of these vibrating rings so you can bring me even more pleasure when we make love," and he hears "You're not adequate, your penis isn't adequate, you can't make me come, I want another man in our bed," it can help to look for toy information together.

Here are some of my favorites, listed in alphabetical order.

BABELAND

www.babeland.com

Formerly Toys in Babeland, this store is very women-friendly and women-focused, although it also carries products for men. A wealth of how-to articles cover everything from anal sex to same-sex sex to what toys are made of. If you live in Seattle, New York, or Los Angeles, check out the events calendar for a wonderful range of hands-on classes.

COME AS YOU ARE

www.comeasyouare.com

Canada, this is one of your best natural resources. The sex educators here do everything right: They hand-select the best products, they offer classes and education that go far beyond the basics, and they devote an entire section of the website to sex and disability. This ranges from allergies to motor control and mobility to issues with decreased or increased sensation. The section recommends specific products and also tells you how to adapt devices you already have, along with tips for enjoying and enhancing your sexuality even as you cope with pain, illness, injury, or impairment.

EXTREME RESTRAINTS

www.extremerestraints.com

This is to BDSM what Sephora.com is to makeup. It has everything, and its online store shows everything too. This is not a site you can sneak-browse at work or with the kids in the room unless you are prepared to do a *lot* of explaining.

FREDDY AND EDDY

www.freddyandeddy.com

Freddy and Eddy started as a toy review site for couples of all persuasions before bowing to audience demands to start their own store. Now they are renowned for their beautiful showrooms in Los Angeles (and if the photos on the website don't get you searching Southwest.com for a cheap trip out, nothing will), as well as for their ability to find the best toys for two. "You hot single folks will probably find most of our stuff boring," they say, but I've not found that to be the case.

GOOD VIBRATIONS

www.goodvibes.com

Good Vibrations is not just a store, it's a university, a museum, and a culture. One of the first to bring toys out of the smut shack, it is all-inclusive: all genders, orientations, preferences, and everything in between. The Antique Vibrator Museum is an eye-opening journey through the liberation of female sexual pleasure, while events like the annual amateur erotic film competition and interviews with luminaries like Margaret Cho create a community that lasts

LET'S GET PHYSICAL—ER, POLITICAL

Some states prohibit the marketing, production, or sale of "devices intended to stimulate the human genitals." Before you order from an online store, make sure they deliver to your state. If they don't, you can still order "back massagers" from The Sharper Image or any health-related store. That limits your options quite a bit, but it's better than nothing. And while you're waiting for it to arrive, write your elected officials and demand they stop thinking so much about your sex lives and get their laws out of your bedroom. Why is it their business what you do with your genitals? They claim they are "protecting the children" by keeping adult stores out of the state, but all they're doing is reinforcing the idea that women are not entitled to sexual pleasure, that only "bad" people use sex toys, and that teenagers should develop shame around sex as quickly as possible in order to be "good" citizens.

long after your shiny new vibrator arrives in the mail. Stores in San Francisco, Berkeley, and Boston host regular workshops and events.

JT'S STOCKROOM

www.stockroom.com

Stockroom was very probably the first sex-toy store to start on the Internet—Joel Tucker founded it in the early 1990s, using his university's email system to send out text-only catalogs. Stockroom focuses on beautiful, well-crafted utensils for your kinkier side. There's something here for everyone: floggers and crops, restraints and clamps, fetish clothing and medical-grade instruments. The site doesn't delve into how-to, but it does offer an online fetish movie theater.

ORGASM ARMY

www.orgasmarmy.com

People from all over the world come to this community site to review toys, condoms, lubes, and other sex products—including intimate shave creams, herbal erection tablets, and aromatherapy for lovers. If you find something you like, a direct link takes you to the fabulous UK-based LoveHoney store.

Part II:

Flirting

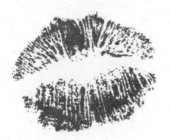

Once we get more comfortable with the realization that the Internet is not entirely composed of pedophiles and porn addicts, we often cannot help ourselves: We have to participate.

Flirting is probably one of the top five most popular online activities. Something about the medium brings out that side of us. If you've ever accidentally flirted with a coworker over the company instant message account, you know the lure. Writing taps into that part of us that journals—and online, most of the time, the journal writes back.

Of course, we're not just flirting with strangers and new friends. All of our communication devices give us new ways to flirt with our partners. You've probably already noticed that no matter how long you've known someone, you learn another side when you begin to interact in text. You might find your lover has a fine ear for puns that he or she hides in polite company. You both might be more bold in your innuendo when you're not face to face.

One advantage to online or mobile flirting is that you can do it while you're doing something else: working, paying the bills, researching a term paper. You can flirt with several people at once, in public and private, with or without their knowing about the others. (It's fair: They don't have to tell you who else they might be wooing.)

Honing your flirting skills online improves your confidence and your wordplay offline, whether you're in a relationship or dating or too busy for anything offline. This section contains lessons for women who want to participate in online sexuality without committing to anything.

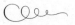

How to Find an Adult Community With Nice, Smart People in It

HOT!

You've heard that anyone can venture online, anytime, day or night, and get swept into a sexual experience so profound she neglects family, friends, and work to spend time on the computer. You've also heard that the Internet is a seething pit of pedophiles, social outcasts, and perverts, and that no self-respecting woman would ever look beyond weather forecasts, driving directions, and iVillage.

Forget what you've heard. The Internet is people, in all our variety, and you have almost total control over who you spend time with while you're online.

Part of the appeal of adult communities is the freedom to let your hair down and say just about anything. Flirt as explicitly as you want, tell raunchy jokes, dress yourself or your avatar in sexy outfits—whether or not you want to have cybersex.

That freedom is most comfortable when you trust the core community, the small group of regulars who care about the quality of the space and who bond with one another as friends and lovers. It's worth putting some effort into finding a place where you belong.

SHOULD I PAY FOR IT?

Pros

★ Most likely everyone in the adult community is an adult.

★ Everyone is invested in keeping the community strong and fun.

★ Active moderators keep the spammers and hecklers out.

Cons

★ You might have to use a credit card to verify your age and pay for the membership.

★ If you leave, you have to remember to cancel.

★ It costs money, of course. Not much, but some.

The more "barriers to entry," the more likely you will find a solid community. People who are making the extra effort to interact in 3D worlds or webcam chat rooms—especially if they are paying for the privilege—tend to be rather fierce about keeping it worth their while, kicking out the jerks and protecting the regulars. (I'm not saying you won't find a good community for free; it just might take longer to find it.)

To start your search, think about the frustrations you might encounter with various digital environments. Is your Internet connection fast enough to handle several webcam video streams at once? Does your computer have enough oomph to handle the graphics and audio of a 3D world or video game? Are you going to be sneaking into the community from work?

BUT WHAT ABOUT
PROTECTING THE CHILDREN?

If the adult community does not require you to assert that you are of legal age, skip it. While it's true that some teenagers will lie about their age, at least with an age check you know minors won't accidentally stumble into it. And it's very hard for a teenager to masquerade as an adult. If you suspect you're talking to an underage person, let the moderator know. Meanwhile, if you're worried too much about whether youth might be lurking in the adult space, stick with premium services and webcams.

Answering those questions will help you figure out whether you should stick with classic text chat rooms or join the rest of the early adopters in building the next generation of cyberspace.

How to Be Nice to Everyone,
Even If They Don't Deserve It

 HOT!

Alas, not everyone in online communities is charming, intelligent, or delightful to be around. In fact the Internet is notorious for giving people a safe, anonymous place to mouth off, snark, rant, insult, and generally act like the spoiled, selfish center of the universe they wish they were.

If you have a blog, you've seen this first hand. If you've been blogging for a while, you've learned to ignore it. (Just remember, every "flame"—an angry, inflammatory comment a reader posts to your blog—is another pageview for you, if you're tracking your traffic.)

The nice thing about adult communities is that people really are there to share the love. Most of the time, these communities are private enough that you don't get the casual haters. Unfortunately, it means that people who infiltrate the community on purpose to troll have enough time on their hands to do so. But in a good community, people are quick to close ranks and kick out the outright jerks.

The best thing you can do to protect your good time is to be universally civil. You don't have to—and you won't—like everyone in any community you become part of, but as your mom says, if you can't say something nice, don't say anything at all. It profits no one to respond to the bait, difficult as it is to ignore.

Some other tips for being nice to everyone:

★ Use the Block or Ignore commands of whatever community tool you're using. If you change your mind later, you can always remove them from the blacklist.

★ Use "please" and "thank you" and "good morning" and other friendly phrases to show your good intentions.

★ Emoticons are your friends. Smiles, winks, and grins help other people understand your intentions so they don't have to try to interpret your mood from your words.

★ Chatspeak is another way to give other people clues. An "lol" (laugh out loud) or "j/k" (just kidding) helps them know you're being playful.

★ Remember that not everyone knows English as a first language, so many clichés and sayings won't make sense to all of your companions. This can be a fun opportunity to flirt and get to know someone better as you try to explain what you meant; they might also offer equivalent expressions in their native tongues.

★ If you're a regular in an adult community, presumably you go there for fun. It's more fun for everyone when each person makes the effort to give others the benefit of the doubt. If you're feeling down or irritated, say so, and give your friends a chance to help cheer you up—and don't resist them when they do.

★ If you find that you're more often frustrated than happy to be there, move on. Communities naturally grow and split and reform and split again. You can remain in touch with the people you are closest to through other means, or even take them with you to find or start a new hangout. But don't set yourself up for misery by being unable to let go of a place that's gone bad.

How to Compose
Erotic Email

HOTTER!

While English teachers groan and bemoan the supposedly "lost art" of letter writing, email has helped millions of women discover their inner Anaïs Nins and Pat Califias. (Hey, they didn't call it "Hotmail" for nothing.) It's true that typing and sending an email takes less time than writing by hand and sealing and stamping envelopes. But as anyone who has ever tried to express love, longing, and lust with mere words can tell you, the composition process is just as painful as ever.

It's worth it though. And you don't have to be a professional writer or award-winning author to tingle your lover's toes. These tips will have you crafting heart-pounding, blood-roaring prose so hot, your English teacher will forget that you didn't write it out by hand.

★ Present tense works especially well, as it puts your lover immediately into the story: *I wrap my arms around you, drawing you closer to me with each breath. Your pulse pounds in your throat; I can feel your heartbeat against my breasts.*

★ Weave in details from your shared history to add authenticity and show your lover that you cherish the memories. For example, mention music from an artist you've seen in concert, set the scene in a familiar location, or include a favorite toy: *On the iPod, Lyle Lovett sings mournfully of North Dakota while the storm rages outside. It reminds me of a story you told me once, of when you were a child and your family was stuck in a blizzard, and you stayed up all night playing board games and drinking hot chocolate. I see the child you were in the gleam in your eyes now, and each time the lightning flashes and you grin, making faces at me in the sudden light.*

★ Fantasy is fair game. If you can imagine it, you can write it—even if your body can't do it. Email erotica can involve exotic destinations, improbable positions, impossible feats of stamina and stimulations, winged angel lovers from space: *It has been a long time since I have seen you in your other form, your pelt thick and warm, your paws the size of dinner plates. We are more than lovers, we are mates, bound body and soul not only by love but by the secret we share. I stroke your fur gently as you gaze at me through your lupine eyes—and then you slowly extend the full length of your tongue, suggestive and bold, curling just the tip and drawing your lips back in a feral grin. I catch my breath as desire surges through my center, wanting to laugh but mesmerized by the grace of your movement. In our other forms, we have no words and so we speak with our bodies, and that is the truest language of all.*

★ Every erotica or porn author will tell you that the surest sign that you've written something hot is that it turns you on as you're writing, but sometimes that's simply not practical. It's downright awkward to be writing a personal email at work and realizing that you're late for a meeting—and now you're ready to hump a fire hydrant. Meanwhile, your lover is receiving this email at work too. It's not necessary to set yourselves ablaze every time; a small spark you can fan into a fire later is plenty.

★ Even if you're just dashing off a quickie to let your lover know you're hot for them, try to engage the senses. Involve smells, tastes, textures, sounds, what things look like, how you feel, how you respond. Even porn stories don't just list a series of actions (he touched, she sucked, he penetrated, they came). What sets erotic email apart from erotic short stories is that it's all about your lover(s) and you, which means it's a perfect vehicle for showing your appreciation for their talents, showing things you'd like to do, and giving them a window into your mind if you've been in a rut of work–kids–chores–sleep–repeat for a while.

How to Make Erotic Art with Cell Phones

HOTTER!

Cell phone cameras have been around for ten years now, and they've come a long way from the grainy thumbnails they produced in the beginning. They are indispensable for long-distance lovers, and they're a fun way to express yourself when words simply won't do.

★ Think holistically. The key here is to expand your—and your lover's—idea of what constitutes an "erotic" body part. Nipples and genitals are obvious, and by all means, share. Yet you can get a lot more creative with unexpected parts of your body. The inside of an elbow, the back of a knee, the hollow beneath an anklebone all have their own interest. Over time you can map the topography of each other's bodies and discover beautiful, sensual, kissable places you never noticed before.

★ A cell phone is immediate, so it's easy to experiment with angles and distances until you find the shots that please you the most. A hand mirror can help you see what's on the display when you're aiming the lens at yourself.

★ Mirrors are also great for adding interest to the pictures. I once took a picture of my freshly shaven coochie by lying on my bed, putting my heels on the wall, and angling the mirror between my thighs. I got a great picture of my legs, the headboard, and part of my belly—plus a bit of hoo-hoo in the mirror that one might not notice at first glance.

★ Play "name this curve."

★ If you have the time, use glitter, makeup, body paint, stencils, or henna dye on the body parts that are taking center stage that day.

> This is one of those activities that combines the thrill of the uninhibited with the power of trust. But it's not going to hurt anything to keep your face out of the pictures, either. In fact, unless you don't care if these pictures go beyond the recipient either by accident or on purpose, I'd advise against including your face in any picture that involves nudity.

★ At the office, you can snap pictures of your skirt hem, your stocking-clad toes, your collarbone barely visible under a silk shell.

★ If your phone has a self-timer, use it to set up more elaborate shots. A three- to ten-second delay is plenty of time to stand on your head, swing from the chandelier, or arrange your stockings and handcuff your other wrist to the bedpost before the image is captured.

★ I prefer to send cell snapshots to my lover's email rather than to his phone. This allows me to use a higher resolution and a larger picture size, and it means the pictures aren't stored on his phone, where his boss or child might accidentally come across it.

★ Some phones have black-and-white or sepia modes that let you add a vintage flavor to your work of art.

★ Trot out that lingerie you don't wear anymore and take close-ups of the lace over your breast, the satin along your hip, or any other part that looks particularly good. The advantage here is you get the flavor of the sexy clothing, even if it's worn out, doesn't fit anymore, or smells like the cat napped on it.

How to Get Phone Alerts in an Exotic Place

HOTTEST!

Yes, you can leave your phone on vibrate and slip it into a pocket. You can even leave it on silent and check it obsessively for love texts. Or you can buy a cheap novelty item that finally explains where we got the expression "give me a buzz."

Some of these products are not likely to bring you to orgasm without some focused, intentional use, but they certainly add dimension to phone alerts!

THE TOY

The Toy is a Bluetooth-enabled vibrator that responds to incoming text messages, and since it does a different motion for every character in the message, you might want to make sure your lover has time for an extended conversation. Once you get it paired with your phone (which admittedly can be a bit of a process), you wear it inside your vagina like a giant plastic tampon and then await your swain's epistles. The moisture-proof antenna acts as a removal cord.

The Toy only responds to messages that begin with a special code, so don't worry about it going off for anyone you haven't authorized to trigger it. And while it doesn't touch the clitoris, I was surprised at how enjoyable the sensation is. It didn't fall out or leave me numb, nor did it make my muscles sore—even though I wore it all day as part of my test.

VIBRAEXCITER

The VibraExciter is a small bullet vibrator that slips easily inside your panties and plugs into a receiver that clips to your belt or fits in a pocket. It responds to the radio frequencies of cell phone transmissions, so any text message or call within a certain range will set it off, and *bzzzzzzz*—you are left in no doubt that someone is calling you (or someone near you). It's a lightweight novelty that probably won't last as long as The Toy, but it also costs significantly less, making it a fun gift for a bachelorette party and a low-commitment step into the world of secretly using sex toys in public.

BODITALK

The BodiTalk, created by the people who brought you the OhMiBod audio vibrator, begins to vibrate when you receive or place a call with your mobile phone. It then continues to rev for the duration of the call (unless you talk so long your battery gives out before your voice does). Unlike the other two devices listed here, it's not designed for use in public places, being rather large for hiding in your pants. But don't let me stop you—far be it for me to tell you where you can and can't put it. As long as you use it safely (it's not designed for anal penetration), you're all good.

How to Meet an International Superstud or Sex Kitten

HOTTER!

Longing for a little British accent to go with your bangers and mash as you travel to the UK? Or perhaps you just really want to meet a hottie to take as a date to your friend's wedding in Italy. Meeting an international superstud or sex kitten can be as simple as logging on to the right site.

When one of my friends decided to travel to Ireland for a few weeks, she knew that it would be a heck of a lot more fun to have the genuine article serenading her in a pub . . . so she hit MySpace.com and did a search for Irish babes. They were surprisingly open to squiring around an American for a week or so, promising to hit everything from the fanciest tavern to the most casual dive.

It goes without saying that pubs were the logical choice for figuring out if Guinness really does taste better in Ireland. (It does.) And while her guide didn't end up being the love of her life, he certainly added a bit of *craic* to the party.

Other places to meet traveling companions:

SECOND LIFE

Create your own avatar and let loose in a virtual global community. With a large majority of non-American members (at press time, the population was

DATING WITHOUT BORDERS

Dating internationally can be exciting, romantic, and expensive, but as you know from your friend of a friend who is marrying the guy she met on the plane, on vacation, or from another country, stranger things have happened.

Typically, Australians, Canadians, and Germans are the most prolific travelers. Taking advantage of generous leave times and a culture geared toward embracing exploration, you will meet friendly and generous folks from these parts of the world everywhere you go. They are fantastic about including you into the group and introducing you to even more new people. Learn a few phrases in other languages to meet the locals, but find the traveling Aussie to make a new drinking partner and possibly find a little romance.

60 percent European), the only limits to meeting someone new are your own adventurous parameters.

LOCAL BARS THAT CATER TO AN INTERNATIONAL SET

Check www.yelp.com, http://Citysearch.com, and local nightlife guides from your alternative weekly papers for the hip hangouts. If you live near a university, check its website for hints of how to connect with students from other lands.

AIRPLANES

You have at least seven hours of time and an entire flight of people. You'd be

CROSS-CULTURAL COMMUNICATION

Forget that you are American, and open your mind to understanding that another culture may find our political situation hilarious.

There are many "quick start" books for communicating cross-culturally. One friend of mine took a book about dirty Italian phrases with her to Italy and had every bartender write updates in the margins. ("That way I knew when a man was commenting on my bodacious tatas," she says. "Asking them to write in my book worked like a charm as a pickup line too.")

Use those expressive eyes that you have been practicing on the webcam. Sometimes it takes no words to communicate what you are thinking if you know how to utilize those peepers.

When desperate, pull up Altavista's free language translation site and plug in the phrase you need translated into English. Just remember that the software is far from perfect, so the translation should be taken as a literal description that might need some additional explaining.

surprised by how many people take advantage of the opportunity to strike up friendships on the trip over. To exert some control over who you sit with, register at AirTroductions.com—a kind of social networking site for frequent travelers—and see who else is going with you.

INTERNATIONAL TRAVEL WEBSITES FOR LOCAL TRAVELERS

Scour travel sites from other countries to see where they recommend their citizens visit, and book your next international trip there. The British Virgin Islands cater to a huge influx of European travelers every August.

ONLINE BUDDIES' RECOMMENDATIONS

Let your online buddies guide you to where you can stay, and favor small, intimate settings like bed-and-breakfasts and hostels. These foster interaction among guests in a way the big hotels don't. If you know your buddies well, you can even stay with them, although it's best to spend at least the first night in a neutral place, such as your reserved lodging. Check the cancellation policies so you know how much refund or cost savings to expect if you end up going home to stay with your friend's mother instead.

ONLINE DATING SERVICES

Match.com, www.RSVP.com.au, Adult Friend Finder, eHarmony, and iFriends all provide search tools to find people in other parts of the world. Set up an online profile to fish for some people to meet while you are visiting.

How to Analyze
a Personal Ad

 HOT!

What started as a fairly marginalized and private concept for the advanced cyber few of the early '90s has mainstreamed itself now as one of the primary ways to meet your next lover. The sheer number of books about online dating—specifically online dating, not just dating books in general—goes to show you that just because something is mainstream doesn't mean it's easy to find overnight success. Online dating may not be as simple as it seems. Or, at least, enough people seem to think they have discovered the secret trick to finding the perfect person online and want to make lots of money writing a book to lead others in search of the Holy Grail.

After all these years, I'm not sure there is a secret trick or a Holy Grail. Relationships are relationships no matter where you go, and let's face it: Dating is kind of silly, anyway. I've always felt that the key to successful dating is to keep your sense of humor and not take it or yourself too seriously.

A quick recap of the premise of online dating:

★ The profile writer says a little bit about him- or herself, and then you have to accept the role of "code cracker." Does "quirky" mean "unbearably weird"? Does "I like independent women" mean "I don't have time for a girlfriend"?

Does "money not important" mean "need sugar mama"? Does "spiritual but not religious" mean "I don't know what I believe, so don't ask," or "I am a spiritual guru who has found the new path to enlightenment"?

★ The profile reader scans for red flags and deal breakers, weighs them against how hot the picture is, and determines whether to contact the person.

★ The profile writer gets a delightful number of emails, signifying that a way to online Mecca has been found. If the inbox comes up dry, the writer either revamps and tries to determine the offending lines, delights in his or her individuality, or hits Amazon.com to buy the aforementioned online dating advice books.

★ An in-person date ensues—or at least some hot and heavy cyber communication.

★ Once you take things to flesh and blood, try not to default back into outdated modes of dating. You're beyond "The Rules"—try just acting like adult people who respect and like each other, and grow from there.

We can't apply one set of rules against all personal ads. But these tips can help you figure out whether you want to make contact.

Look for stock phrases. If an ad contains too many things along the lines of "likes children and puppies, long walks at sunset," watch for a possible faker or just an extremely boring person whose mom wrote their ad.

Watch for language aimed specifically for or against one segment of the population, and make sure you are okay with their criteria. For example, "I like skinny actress types who want to be stay-at-home moms and serve as arm candy at my next black tie function. If people tell you that you weigh more wet, you are the girl for me!" Just a guess, but this writer has a thing for unreality and really will want to see if you weigh more wet before asking for another date.

Look at the complete picture the person presents. If they list a job and hobbies that effectively tie them up every work day and all day Saturday and Sunday on the golf course, know that unless you work where they work or play how they play, you are likely to have conflicting schedules, at least until that mad love hits.

Ask for clarification on things that may seem obvious if you are uncertain about word usage. For example, "I must have someone with conservative sexual needs." This can be taken to mean anything from "I don't want it very often, and when I do, it needs to be of the vanilla variety," to "I am willing to do anything between two consenting adults but don't want to share you with anyone else." Either, both, or neither may be acceptable to you, but what a bummer if you took it to mean the first when it was really the latter!

If the pictures look old (dated styles, baby-face look, grainy, scanned picture instead of digital), they probably are old. And if the person looks slightly familiar in that "gorgeous, but looks familiar" kind of way, you may be well served to peruse the latest Abercrombie catalog. If the picture looks professional, you may have a scammer on your hands, unless the person *is* a model. (Hey, it happens, particularly in Los Angeles and New York. Those guys have a hard time meeting people who take them seriously, and the online realm gives them a chance to connect as people first and bodies second. Really.)

How to Craft a Personal Ad That Truly Expresses Who You Are

 HOT!

Most people surf through tens if not hundreds of profiles every time they search a dating site. If you sound like everyone else, you are going to be treated like everyone else.

Stop the boredom! There are tons of articles about writing the perfect profile on sites like Yahoo Personals, Match.com, and Cupid.com—and each one is slanted toward the profiles of the particular dating service. Online dating expert Evan Marc Katz offers advice and sample profile makeovers in his e-newsletter. (You can get the full scoop at www.evanmarckatz.com.) Many, many books exist on the subject if you want to get obsessive about it.

These ten tips should get you started down the right path.

★ Know your audience, and speak to them. Search for the profiles of your target audience, and match your language to theirs. The subtle mimicking of words and ideas will attract the people who think the way you like.

★ Understand the site you are using. For example, in adult dating networks like AdultFriendFinder.com, you can get explicitly sexual and kinky in your text (although not as much so in your photos) without violating the terms of service. At Match.com, however, you'll find a more general audience, some of whom are likely to flag you for "offensive material" if you get too raunchy, ensuring that your profile never gets found. (Know thy screeners, as well as thy audience!)

★ Show, don't tell. Use your photos to paint the picture of a dog-loving, REI-shopping, adventurous world traveler. Instead of just putting in the stock headshots, post the picture of you standing on the Great Wall of China with your friends, or rolling in the mud with your Great Dane. But don't PhotoShop yourself onto a backdrop. One day, someone will ask you about that trip, and making up a good story can be tricky, especially if you've attracted a true world traveler with your pictures.

★ Stop with the clichés! Who cares if you are "fun-loving," "funny" and "physically fit?" Blah. Everyone says that. Try instead: "My trainer has become one of my best friends—not only do we work out together 3x a week, but we visit the Saxon Pub at least once a month to see our favorite local guitarist hit some new riffs." See . . . fun and fit in the same sentence.

★ Be funny instead of saying you are funny. Yes, we know that men don't tend to list "sense of humor" as high on their must-have lists as women do, but if you can elicit a laugh, you might catch the attention of someone who shares your quirky outlook on life. Most people will contact a person they feel a connection with, or a person who makes them feel happy. This may not apply to the brooding artists of the world, but then again, your dark-side-of-the-moon commentary might just attract the neighbor who secretly listens to you practicing your guitar on the back step at night. You just never know.

★ Yes, sex sells . . . but again, know your audience. If you really are trying to find a quality connection, leave the sex for later. Otherwise, you're likely to be overwhelmed with come-ons from men you have no interest in, and you could miss a good one in the flood. When you meet—ya either got it or ya don't. Leave it under wraps until you actually want to act on it. If you are on a site where hookups are the primary focus, then sex away, and revel in the power of free speech.

★ Leave the defensiveness, posturing, and negativity at the door. For example, if a man feels like you're dissing his entire sex before you even meet him, he's going to pass on by. Yes, as adults, most of us have had bad experiences. Talk to your therapist about it, but don't use your online profile to try to change the world.

★ Pack your words tightly. Read through your completed profile and take out any filler. For example: "I like to run. I would love to find someone who wants to run with me. Running in the morning is particularly wonderful. I run marathons occasionally as well, and I am a member of the local running group. I make running a boring topic by going on and on like this indefinitely, and it's all I know how to talk about." If you lose a reader before they even get a paragraph in, they aren't going to want to hear what you have to say in person either. Try instead, "If you are looking for a marathoner who loves seeing the first blush of dawn over the water . . . let's meet up for a jog on the beach before work and see if we can make it all the way to the breakfast taco stand and back." I'm not even a runner, and that sounds fun to me.

★ Don't talk about your exes on your profile. Obvious? Yes. So why do so many people do it? And why do they post photos of themselves with their old flames present or badly cropped out? As far as your profile content is concerned—you have no exes, your ex-boyfriend is not crazy, and you think dating is just a world of incredible possibilities.

★ Spell check. Please, please, please. And especially don't misspell the word "intelligent." I've seen it happen. Multiple times. It's pretty hard to redeem that one.

How to Tell Whether You Are Connectivity Compatible

HOTTER!

Those who give good word have the best chance of attracting women online, whether they're writing a personal ad, flirting mildly over email, or chatting in an adult room.

But e-courtship creates the expectation that you will continue to regale each other with daily (at least!) epistles in email, instant messages, and text messages long after your relationship has solidified. And problems can arise when one party craves the online interaction while the other can't wait to dispense with it and engage solely in person.

I personally have a high desire for Internet intimacy. It doesn't have to be sexual (well, not all the time), but it has to be something: an email about his day, a new joke, an hour of instant messaging before (or from) bed.

I've also found that if a man doesn't interest me online, he doesn't interest me offline either. I can't get to know the whole person without email or instant messaging. We're different in our online writing—funnier, braver, more intimate. I want to know that side of my lover, and I really notice its lack when it's missing.

For anyone who has invested a lot of time and thought into email love letters, or who has reveled in the nakedness of late-night instant messaging, dropping those elements from the relationship is the modern update to "You don't bring me flowers anymore."

Then there's the other side. You might be the one who's not interested in connectivity. You might be over it now that you're together, in person. You might not have been that interested to begin with but went along when that was how you were getting to know one another.

During courtship, think about how involved your new flame is in the connectivity side of things. Do you send a dozen emails for every one you get back? Are you always glancing at your IM list, hoping to see that special someone pop up? Are you annoyed that he or she is running your cell phone bill up with endless text messages? If it's already a burden, are you sure you want to pursue this relationship?

If you are radically different in your connectivity preferences, yet committed to the relationship, you can fill the void by chatting with your friends instead. Then treasure every missive from your lover, even if it's just a text message that says "omw" (on my way).

Or, if you're wondering why your partner is spending so much time on the computer, it might simply be that you're not providing as many virtual touches as you could be. And it's likely they aren't seeking a new relationship or a cyber affair—it may just be that it hasn't occurred to the blockhead to ask you to IM once in a while.

It doesn't matter where on the spectrum you fall, as long as you and your partner find the right balance so that no one feels overwhelmed and no one feels neglected.

How to Flirt with Anyone Online

HOTTER!

Flirting online is one of my favorite side activities. It alleviates the solitude of working from home and gives me a reason to be at my computer that's not entirely work-related.

One of the joys of the Internet is you can flirt with any adult of any gender, sex, and sexual preference without causing anyone undue distress. In some contexts, it's simply the polite thing to do.

Now, I recognize that flirting is an individual thing, and this lesson is a general one. But I've been flirting online since 1994 (right, Ron?), and I lost count long ago of all the playmates I've been blessed with in my cyberlife. And I can tell you with confidence that some principles apply across all media, whether you're in a highly immersive 3D environment or a text-only message board.

Flirting online encompasses a wide range of communications, from a gentle compliment to explicitly erotic requests. Unless we're on webcam, we don't have body language cues like eye contact, hair twirling, or parting our lips to help us set the right tone, and if we're in a group situation, we have the additional challenge of making sure our targets know we're talking to them.

Like we do in the rest of our lives, we get along best online if we act in a way that's appropriate to our environments. I wouldn't whip out the same lexicon in a professional forum that I would in a naked dance party at a virtual club. Any flirting I do outside of a designated adult environment, I make sure to keep within the bounds of things I would say at a casual after-work gathering with fun coworkers.

In an adult environment though, look out. This is where you can use language you can't whip out anywhere else. Tell raunchy jokes, mention breasts and pussies, praise men's cocks and women's dancing, and remember their preferences from past conversations, and you'll be the most popular gal in the room.

In online dating contexts, I suggest taking a middle ground. These are folks you're likely to meet in person, and you don't want to set expectations too soon. Where you might have an extended punwar on the concept of "penis" in an adult chat room, in an IM session with a prospective date, you should probably stick to less intimate subjects.

The absence of body language means you have to use your words, and if you can find others who like using their words, online flirting is the hottest flirting you're going to get anywhere. You can be direct and explicit or coy and demure, as long as you are honest in your interest and willing to let others have their say too—even if they don't type as fast as you do.

If you're just wanting to flirt and not looking for anything more, it's best to mention that periodically in the public room so newcomers know not to pester you. Flirting equally with everyone in the room who participates in the general conversation also helps manage both expectations (no one will expect you to meet them in private, although many will ask) and emotions (you won't get overly attached to just one and threaten any existing relationships).

The secret to successful flirting online is no different from any other type of relationship building. If you respect their sexual desires and embrace them enthusiastically, they will want to engage with you. You don't have their genitals in your face, so their bodily plumbing ceases to matter. You can engage with people at face value, as they present themselves, and learn how your own communication style changes based on other people's genders and orientations.

How to Find a
Dinner Date by Tonight

HOTTER!

If you want to go out to dinner with a date tonight, probably the first order of business is to let go of expectations and lower your standards. I don't mean go out with someone who repulses you—but don't expect to assess this person in terms of lifelong relationships.

It's just dinner.

In multiple cities across the North America, Craigslist holds a strong local online presence, and its personals are known for fostering an "instant gratification" atmosphere. The only downside is that they don't have that nifty little "online now" icon to shortcut the search for someone who could start making plans with you right this minute.

Local is key for instadating. Look for sites that are geographically focused, like www.austinsingles.org, http://outinatlanta.com, online newspapers, and so on. You can also take a large dating site and narrow your search results to a 5- or 10-mile radius. Give priority to the person who is "online now," chat for half hour an or so to make sure he or she is not going to bore you to death, and then arrange to meet for dinner.

WHAT DO WE *NOT* TALK ABOUT?

★ Politics

★ Religion

★ Family

★ How many kids we want

★ Sex

★ Ex flames

Your results will vary, since your main search criteria is someone who is online now and available tonight, not someone who is the best mate for you in all the world. The person might be boring or obnoxious. The date might be a lot of fun but not go anywhere.

Be very specific that you're looking for a dinner date; that you will pay your own way and that you're not propositioning for a hookup. Surprise chemistry is always fun, but just in case that chemistry only goes one way, set up the expectations in advance so you can make a graceful exit if needed. Don't forget to follow all the safety procedures that you normally would for a date with a stranger. Visit any online dating or sex worker information site for a list of standard precautions, such as meeting in a public venue and arranging to call a friend to check in at a particular time.

The idea here is to be fun and funny and spontaneous, to talk about the randomness of it all, and to enjoy that little endorphin rush that comes from a surprise at the end of your day. You can afford to keep it light and simple, because it's just dinner, and if you don't like your date, you can cut it short.

ARE YOU SURE IT'S JUST DINNER?

I think it's a good idea not to let "just dinner" turn into a hookup (that is, casual sex or a one-night stand). That trains your dates to think "just dinner" means "just dinner and then the oral sex," which sounds wonderful to me but might be a shock to the next girl. It also lets you get away with fooling yourself about your own motives.

If you are saying "dinner" but meaning "sex," listen to yourself. There's nothing wrong with that—just be honest (with yourself and with your dates) about what you really want.

Keep total control by paying your own way, driving yourself, and meeting somewhere outside your usual circle.

This approach also serves the shy, nervous, or obsessively analytical dater by decreasing the amount of time you have to obsess about the situation. You make the date, and a few hours later, you are on it.

If you are one of the "must buy a new outfit for a new date" kind of gals, you may struggle with this one—unless you have a personal shopper on call who can deliver the latest and greatest to your door within hours.

If that surprise chemistry takes you hostage and it turns into a hookup, don't kick yourself over it. If you hit it off that much you can always make another date—this time for breakfast!

How to Seduce Someone
Using Gadgets You
Already Have in Your Purse

 HOTTEST!

The New York Times rocked the establishment in late 2006 when it reported that when it comes to romantic gifts, most women would rather receive a big-screen television than diamond jewelry. (Raise your hand if this surprised you.) I don't know why we persist in thinking of gadgets as a man's world; women are just as interested in having the gear to support our lifestyles.

Gear, like sex, is highly personal. I like my LG 9900 cell phone, which opens up to expose a QWERTY keyboard for text messaging and email. It's heavier than a BlackBerry or Sidekick, and its keys are farther apart and require a stronger press. This works for me—but others can't stand the thought of carrying such a brick around in their pockets or purses.

But gear is one of the advantages we have over our ancestresses. Our everyday gadgets, like PDAs and cell phones and MP3 players, have some surprising new applications.

We're human. The first thing we do with any new technology is figure out how to have sex with it. These tips will help you work your gear the way a burlesque dancer works her feathers.

★ Use your cell phone to send your partner an erotic text message, or to leave a sexy voicemail on a phone you know he or she can't answer at the moment.

★ On a date, wait until you are seated and your lover's eyes are on you. Pull your über-cool phone out of your bag, murmuring something about putting it in silent mode. As you handle it, stroke it softly, cup it in your palm, caress the buttons—in other words, hint at your other skills, while pretending to be completely innocent of the effect your graceful motions are having.

★ Snap a picture of your lips, glistening and glossy and slightly parted, and send it with a text message saying you'll be in your lover's bed at 8:00 PM with nothing on but the radio.

★ Whip out that PDA and schedule your next date right in front of your lover. Tell your lover that it's going to be your treat, and that you expect to get laid.

★ Load a slideshow of erotic pictures onto your iPod before your next fancy dinner date. While lingering over your gooey, sensual dessert, hand your lover the iPod and kick off your shoe. Caress your lover's leg under the table while you make soft sensual noises and make oral love to your spoon.

Part III:

Self - Expression

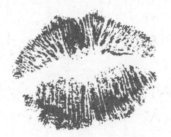

Most women have something to say about love, sex, and relationships. But until fairly recently in history, we could only say it to our closest friends, and even then, only in whispers.

Now we can say our piece to as many people who care to listen. We can say it anonymously, if necessary—a traditional form of female expression. (As Virginia Woolf said, "For most of history, Anonymous was a woman."). We can say it so well and so professionally that we can become Internet famous for it; or we can keep it on a smaller scale.

This section contains lessons for using technology as a platform for your sexual expression, whether it is writing erotica, performing on camera, or creating a 3D avatar.

This is the point of the information age. It's what Internet and mobile technology is all about, and it's what women are good at: sharing, expression, communication, and multitasking, among other things.

How to Be an
Exhibitionist Online

HOTTEST!

One of the fun ways to play online is to learn how to parade around like the sex kitten you know you are. And one of the common consequences is a greater comfort with your body and sensuality in the rest of your life. You might find yourself wiggling more, swaying more, undulating more—and wearing less—in the bedroom, much to your lover's delight.

Exhibitionism isn't just about taking your clothes off though. You can exhibit your sexual self in all kinds of ways—through word and deed—that benefit you in other aspects of your life.

And all it takes is a stroll through newbienudes.com to see that you don't have to be nineteen years old to attract an appreciative audience.

★ Find an outfit you like and practice posing with various cameras—cell phone, pocket, pro, webcam, whatever you have—until you're comfortable with what angles and poses to use.

★ Use language you wouldn't ordinarily. If you're a lady, try out raunchy. If you're not, go high-falutin'. Play with different tones and voices, and see how far you can take it in text. Then learn to do it in voice.

★ Seductive pictures that hint at nudity offer fun with less risk. Don't forget to keep your face out of the photos unless you trust the recipient 150 percent, or unless it doesn't matter if it gets splashed all over the Internet.

★ If you're really shy, stick with feet and ankles in interesting socks and stockings. Or hands. Or elbows.

★ Cell phone cameras and webcams often have that wide-angle effect in which anything close to the lens gets magnified. This offers an opportunity to capture creative images to share online without revealing anything you couldn't show in public. For example, you can make your eyes exotically large and your chin delicately pointed if you hold the phone above and to one side of your face. Or have it zoom in on the curve of your ankle or behind your knee and capture the shape more than the body part.

★ True exhibitionism requires a live audience, so invest in a great webcam and sign up for a premium account at a service like PalTalk. Again, it's common to keep your face out of the picture. Trot out lingerie, sex toys, body paint and any other visually appealing props that turn you on.

★ Bodies in motion are beautiful. Put on some music and dance, and don't worry if it "looks okay"—it does.

How to Publish Your Sexy Story

HOTTER!

"The best thing about writing erotica now is you can do it without your mother-in-law figuring out you're doing it," says Nobilis, an erotica author who generously shared several tips with me for this book.

The first thing, of course, is to learn to write well. (And once you do, keep practicing!) Erotica is not just a sex scene slapped together out of a stack of dirty words. You need a story, with characters who develop and a beginning, middle, and end.

The next is to find a community. Writing is isolating, lonely, and bleak—no one understands writers, and no one but other writers truly gets the agony of it all. (Tee hee.) The Erotic Readers and Writers Association (ERWA) is a good place to start, as is www.asstr.org, the modern incarnation of the alt.sex.stories repository newsgroup. But there are writers' groups all over the web, so don't feel limited to just these.

Short story writers often start with sites like Literotica.com or Storiesonline (http://storiesonline.net), where you can post your stories and get ratings and

WHERE TO LEARN MORE ABOUT EROTICA

Erotica Readers and Writers Association (ERWA)

http://erotica-readers.com

Articles, forums, and critique groups for erotica fans

Nobilis

www.freewebs.com/nobiliserotica

Has a forum where erotica authors exchange tips, news, and encouragement

reviews from the community. This can be a mixed blessing—take it in the spirit of helpfulness.

Nobilis recommends checking ralan.com, a long-time resource for writers, for a directory of other markets for both stories and e-books, and checking ERWA frequently for calls for submissions to anthologies (online and in print).

Writing erotica at the pro or semipro level requires a combination of talent, imagination, persistence, and business savvy. Even erotica doesn't sell itself. In fact, especially erotica, because there's so much of it, and your gem can be buried among a mountain of bad writing. If you want to write erotica for more than posting to a forum, you need to learn how to promote it too. Virtual book signings, helping other writers, doing podcasts and media interviews—all the tricks of self-promotion come into play with erotica as well.

How to Take
Sexy Self-Portraits

HOTTEST!

Cameras are everywhere. Sooner or later, you're going to be caught in a compromising position. Picking your nose as you run a red light. Adjusting your stockings as Google's street-view team cruises by. Handing your phone around the table in a mutual-gadget-admiration moment with a dozen coworkers, only to realize you haven't deleted Those Pictures from the album. (That one actually happened to me. At my day job. Sigh.)

If you can't hide from 'em, you might as well learn to present your best face—or whatever—any time you suspect you're in the crosshairs of an autofocus lens. And like sexual technique, one of the best ways to learn how to pose for other people is to practice on your own first.

A cell phone camera is all you need to get started, although a small digital camera gives you higher quality images. These first shots aren't for sharing, but rather for learning what the digital eye does to you, and for you, from various distances and angles.

★ Look to classic pin-up poses for inspiration. These flatter every body and have an element of tease and sauce that never goes out of style.

★ If you discover a touch of exhibitionism through your experiments, invest in a mobile device with a high-resolution camera and a self-timer.

★ Hold the camera above your face and slightly to the side to emphasize your eyes and cheekbones.

★ Learn to smile without clenching your facial muscles. It feels horribly fake at first, but works well in pictures. Better yet, cultivate a knowing, subtle quirk of the lip that implies you are just seconds from ripping your clothes off and jumping on your lover.

★ Stretch the crown of your head to the sky, don't pull your chin back into your throat, and let your eyelids feel heavy and languorous as you slide your gaze slightly off to one side.

★ Flushed cheeks, wide eyes, and parted lips are signs of sexual arousal in both sexes. You can fake it by pinching your skin, biting your lips, and opening your eyes slightly wider than usual. Too wide and you'll just look surprised or alien, so practice in a mirror until you get the right feel of it.

★ If you look at porn stars' pictures, you'll see they're often throwing their heads back and looking up at the camera. This makes their hair look longer, their eyes look bigger, and their mouths look open in a rounder O. Hint.

★ Lipstick and gloss.

★ Take the picture first thing in the morning, while you're still puffy from sleep. If necessary, fluff up your bedhead to look more tousled, but don't even brush your teeth first. You want to look like you just rolled out of bed after a late night of lovin'. Your self-portrait will be extra sexy if both of those things are true.

How to Share Your Orgasm for the Sake of Art

HOTTEST!

"This may be the most erotic thing you have ever seen, yet the only nudity it contains is from the neck up. That's where people are truly naked," says Beautiful Agony founder GMBill.

Beautiful Agony is a photo and video gallery of people in the throes of orgasm—but showing only their faces. Anyone can submit their "agony" for inclusion on www.beautifulagony.com, assuming they are over eighteen, meet the technical requirements for digital video, and can follow the instructions for contributing their work. If it is accepted, you not only get to participate in one of the more original online forms of sexual expression, you get a small fee and a free month's membership for experiencing other people's orgasms.

At sister site http://ishotmyself.com, women take things up a notch, submitting videos in which they make a statement about nudity, sex, and the Internet, and they take great pleasure in doing so. The criteria here is that you shoot the video yourself—and no cheating with remote controls, you have to keep one hand on the camera at all times—and then submit it (follow the directions!) for inclusion.

If you want to go pro, the third sister site, http://ifeelmyself.com, celebrates the beauty of the female orgasm. This ever-growing collection of video shows more than faces and has the added bonus of being professionally shot in beautiful lighting and sensual settings. Women from all walks of life apply to be filmed masturbating or having partner sex in environments that allow them to live out their fantasies and provide an alternative to the often abrasive, in-your-face nature of mainstream studio porn.

These are just three examples of how women use technology to challenge our traditional ideas of pornography; every participant is doing her (or his!) part to expand our awareness of the erotic. And even if you don't want to take your orgasms quite so public, all three of these communities offer inspiration for making sexy videos to share with your partners!

How to Be an
Audio Erotica Star

HOTTER!

I first encountered audio erotica in 2003, the first time I covered the annual adult entertainment industry trade show for my "Sex Drive" column. Amidst all the flash and glitz was a beautifully appointed booth that looked more suited to Sephora than to Smitty's Smut Shack. The banner said SOUNDS EROTIC, and I stepped up with a grin and asked "What's that?"

Half an hour later, I had an excellent education in aural sex from husband-and-wife team Catherine and Brian Oliver-Smith.

Married with three children and another one the way, the couple had reached a point where they were too tired to transition from working parents by day to passionate lovers by night. They experimented with porn videos, but Catherine found them more tedious than titillating. Reading erotic stories worked better, but it required the reader to look at the words instead of the other person, and you had to stop fondling to turn the page. Yet it was impractical to call upon a third party to read to them while they kissed and caressed each other.

Recording erotic stories to play back in bed solved the problem. Brian and Catherine found that by the end of about seven minutes, their touches and gazes reawakened their bodies even as the story realigned their minds. Realizing that their plight was a common one for other parents, they launched a publishing company to bring this relationship-saver to other couples. They hire professional voice talent and choose stories specifically adapted for listening to, rather than for reading.

You don't have to be a professional to star in your own erotic recordings, although if you plan to publish the results, you need to make sure you have legal rights to the stories and any sound effects you use in your composition. These tips will help you get off to a smooth start.

★ Choose (or write!) a story that turns you on. If you intend to use someone else's story for purposes outside your personal relationship, make sure you have permission from the author first. Look for good writing that flows well when you read it aloud—it will sound different to your ear than when you read it to yourself.

★ Read through the entire story first, and make note of pronunciations you need to practice (or look up), phrases that tie your tongue, and anything that makes you blush or giggle. You can also mark areas where you want to slow down or speed up, drop your voice to a whisper, or add other dramatic touches. You might think you have no problem reading the descriptions, but you'd be surprised at how the most seasoned professional voices can suddenly be embarrassed or experience stage fright.

★ Take your time. Do not rush it. Think of trying for a slow seduction. As with any public speaking, you will think you are speaking way too slowly, and that's about when it is perfect.

★ Whispering all the time is not sexy. Neither is a monotone. Don't be breathy either; it doesn't work as well as you might think. Mix it up a bit by altering the timbre of your voice, speak more loudly, more softly, quicker then slower, breathe a bit heavier at the sex parts (but never through your nose, which sounds horrible on a recording).

★ Drink some water, wear comfortable clothes that allow you to breathe, and don't move around a lot, as a good microphone will pick up the noise. If you move your head around, the sound will be uneven, which is distracting and can ruin the mood for the listener.

If you really get into it and think you might have what it takes to go pro, consider starting a regular podcast!

How to Blog Your Sex Life
Without Getting Dumped

 HOTTER!

"Writing everything there was to write about my relationships online was probably not a good idea, not because 'Now everyone knows,' but because of the way it changed the relationships for myself and for my partners," says Audacia Ray, author of *Naked on the Internet*. "That said, I did learn an immense amount from the blogging."

While I don't have a problem with TMI (too much information), I concede that sex blogging is a literary and emotional minefield. It is also an incredibly powerful tool for self-examination, sexual discovery, and life improvement. And once you get started, the rewards are often worth the risks.

A blog is simply a website created by a fill-in-the-blanks-and-press-Go publishing tool. That ease of publishing frees you up from having to think about the technical so you can get down to business: keeping the chronicle of your sexual journey.

Sex blogs come in many flavors, from fictional tell-alls to intimate diaries of long-term relationships. Many women start blogging as an outlet to express unhappiness or dissatisfaction—and stop blogging months or years later, when they have found some sort of resolution.

Whatever your motivation for blogging about your sex life, these tips help you navigate the treacherous waters until you reach a safe shore of your own.

YOU ARE NOT ANONYMOUS.

You can, and probably should, attempt discretion. You might use a "nom de net" and never mention anyone else by name or even initials (that's what got the Washingtonienne in trouble). Yet if you are writing about your life, details will emerge, and someone, somewhere, will eventually recognize you.

> Losing your anonymity might wreak havoc with your life, but it's not the end of the world if you're a good writer and willing to step into the limelight.

YOUR PARTNER'S EXES WILL READ YOUR BLOG. SO WILL YOURS.

Remember that you're not just exposing your inner self to people you'll never meet.

BLOGGING INSTEAD OF TALKING IS NOT GOOD FOR YOUR RELATIONSHIP.

It's one thing to work something out in your blog and then talk about it with your partner. It's another to discuss an important relationship issue with a bunch of people on the Internet without ever letting your partner have a clue there's something wrong.

BLOG THE GOOD STUFF TOO.

This is especially important if your partner is reading along, but it's also just good blogging: Provide some balance, so when you go deep into working out an issue, you and your readers have perspective.

Abby Lee—This English author blogged anonymously as "Girl with a One-Track Mind," detailing her sex life from the safety of her pseudonym, Abby Lee. Her writing was so good, and her blog so popular, she ended up with a book contract—and never even revealed her name to her publisher, conducting all transactions through her agent. Just before her book hit the stands, a Sunday newspaper outed her, publishing her real name and turning her into what she describes as the "scarlet woman du jour." All she could do was make the best of it and tell herself that at least she was doing her part to challenge old-fashioned views about female sexuality. Now, she's a best-selling author and highly trafficked blogger who speaks regularly about feminism and sexuality—and who still writes some of the hottest sex on the web.

—Jessica Cutler, http://washingtonienne.com—the famous capital hill ingenue who slept with married coworkers and then blogged, often scathingly, about it. She lost her job but gained a million-dollar book deal.

IF YOU'RE BLOGGING, YOUR PARTNER MIGHT BE BLOGGING TOO.

There's some debate about whether it's better to read or ignore each other's blogs. You can hurt each other pretty hard by comments intended to be clever, or comments that felt like simple venting but now archive an unflattering observation for all time. On the other hand, blogging as if your partner is reading forces you to think everything through, and to phrase it honestly and precisely.

How to Look Great on Webcam

HOTTEST!

It's a heady feeling when you have an audience, and you swivel just so, and you see someone catch his or her breath, and suddenly no one can type well because their fingers aren't working right.

Women rule in webcam chat. I'm sorry if that sounds gender-bound or cliché to you. It's just one of those simple sex-tech truths, like cell phones will always garble the connection on the most romantic phrases, and programmers code better with caffeine.

I've found that I have a parakeet approach to my own image and have a hard time wrenching my gaze from the little window that shows me what my webcam is broadcasting. I've spent a lot of time tilting my head this way or that, leaning forward to show cleavage or back to emphasize the curve of my hips, just to get the feel for what works the best for presenting my body in a flattering way.

Even for porn stars, who use actual digital video cameras instead of the $20 cams from RadioShack, the camera eye flattens what you want to stick out and bulges what you want to keep flat. It also shortens you—I am least four inches taller in real life, I'm certain of it—and highlights anything that contrasts with your skin tone, like moles and pimples and veins.

It's especially unkind if the connection burps and freezes the image while you're moving, displaying 20 seconds of "hippo in a tutu" or "is that a potato or your nose" instead of your truly gorgeous self.

Millions of people have at least dipped their well-pedicured toes into webcam chat. The vast majority don't bleach their anuses, remove every last body hair, or spend their working hours naked. The thrill of cam chat is in the shared sexual energy among ordinary people, in starring in your own erotic film, and in awakening or reawakening your sex drive by remembering just how hot you really are.

For me, part of the fun of using a webcam is taking advantage of the visual medium, not just sitting there watching each other typing or masturbating. Here are a few things I've learned from my time in the spotlight.

★ Use a touch of makeup to bring out your features, but don't go overboard. Webcams don't pick up enough detail to make it worth spackling your face like you would for television, and heavy makeup can make you look masked or dead.

★ If you're with a man, ask him to show off his biceps, his legs, his elbows, and/or his face if he's comfortable with that. Or ask for a tour of his room, or for him to hold up his favorite object that's within arm's reach and tell you why he likes it. Many men start their cameras and focus it only on their crotches. This isn't entirely penis-centric on their part; oftentimes they just don't know what women want to see.

SESKA'S STORY

Seska Lee, a sex educator and performer who has eight years of professional experience on webcam, makes love with her husband James every Tuesday evening in front of a chat room audience of 100–150 people.

The shows are an integral part of her relationship, not just a paid performance. She indulges in a ritual beforehand—bath, scrubbing salts, moisturizing, "everything that makes me feel sexy for myself—and looks forward to Tuesday each week.

"Some people don't like scheduling sex, but I don't feel trapped by that. It's where I give myself one hour of 'me time' with my partner; it's very focused, and I really appreciate setting aside that time," she says.

"On the other hand, I like to think about the audience and that I'm on camera, specifically. I have done burlesque—it's fun—but there is something fun about the camera. And this audience that is somewhere else—that's a turn on."

Seska is slim, fit, curvy, and gorgeous, so it surprised me when she said she doesn't always feel her best. But the show—like the sexual intimacy in a strong relationship—must go on.

"If I'm feeling bloated, I wear something that will cover up my tummy so I don't have to worry about sucking it in," she says. And if she doesn't feel sexy inside, her lack of energy will be obvious on camera. "If I don't have to worry about it, I can just focus on the pleasure and what I'm doing," she says.

"I am a more solid, confident sexual person because of the commitment I've made to webcamming. I'm good at the multitasking, and I use both hands."

RECOMMENDED READING

webAffairs, by art professor Show-n-tell

This documentary-style book takes you on a journey through a typical webcam chat experience, from the initial excitement to the final learning experiences. Along the way, you see how the author's participation affected her marriage, the kinds of people you meet in cam rooms, and how different cultures think about sex, exhibitionism, and love on the Internet. The book has a companion art exhibition and website. It's a fascinating project that took more than four years to complete, and I cannot recommend it highly enough.

★ Invest in lighting. Home Depot sells clip-on lamps you can easily set up and take down. Blue light bulbs simulate daylight and help eliminate shadows. ("Shadows are not your friend," says porn star Taylor Wane, who also performs live on webcam. "The more light on you, the better.")

★ If you are in a chair, lean toward the cam to emphasize the curve of the waist and enlarge the bust. Lean away to add shape to the hips; try pressing your knees together or crossing your legs. This also visually shrinks the waist.

★ Have a good time. Your genuine pleasure will shine through and matter more to others than whether you can hook your ankles behind your head.

★ If your connection is stuttered or delayed, use it to add suspense.

★ Don't do anything you wouldn't want frozen or captured on someone's screen. Webcams seem to know when you've picked at a pimple or worse, and they are notorious for seizing up and leaving that image in the chat room.

★ Anything you do on camera can be captured by anyone on the other end, either through screenshots or more sophisticated recording technology. Most people are there for the same reason you are—to have fun and excitement— but it only takes one angry ex or immature dickweed to take a picture and publish it. Given the number of people participating in cam chat, this doesn't happen very often, but that's no consolation if it happens to you. Keeping your face out of the frame, and making sure the camera doesn't pick up any identifying information (like the address label on a bill) is good practice.

★ Accept that when you look good and damn good, that's the reality. When you look like a funhouse mirror, that's the fake stuff. Your body is sexy just the way it is. Believe it, even when you're offline.

★ When you feel sexy, you look sexy; when you look sexy, you feel sexy.

How to Be
a Webcam Girl

HOTTEST!

There's webcam in a chat room for fun, and then there's setting yourself up to go pro—which can also be fun, if you enjoy multiple sexual relationships, masturbation, and theater. I've lost count of how many woman have told me, "Well, I was having so much fun doing it for free, I decided I might as well get paid."

I called Alyssah Simone, one of the top three models at Flirt4Free (http://flirtforfree.com), to find out what it takes to make a living—and a good one—as a cam girl. This is not a comprehensive guide in a single lesson, alas, but these tips will help you get off to a great start.

★ Check out several cam sites to figure out which one most appeals to your sensibilities, schedule and business and technical savvy. Most sites have a "become a broadcaster" link somewhere on the home page where you can learn the technical and performance requirements.

★ Consider how you will brand yourself. Are you demure? Dominant? Trashy? Ladylike? Some women set up different profiles on the same cam site so they can have one identity as a schoolgirl, one as a dominatrix, one as a cheerleader,

> "I really get to interact with these guys, and there are women too. They open themselves up to me. I get to see all those skeletons in their closet. The people I meet! I can't even begin to tell you. So many different people, different stories. And I have access to all of them, right at that moment, all right there in my chat room. I'm a friend, a lover, even sometimes a mother for them. They tell me things they would never tell anyone else."
>
> —Alyssah Simone, professional cam girl

and so on. That helps you build an audience in each context—some of whom will follow you to all your performances, simply because it's you, and others who stop by because of the particular flavor of the show.

★ Not all of your performance time is billable. At Flirt4Free, performers hang out in the community rooms and flirt, chat, and tease with members for free, to entice them into the paid shows.

★ Women who interact with the audience, who ask questions and engage with their fans as people and not just as walking wallets, tend to develop larger followings (and in turn, make more money). This is the classic paradox of sex work: It's not the prettiest girl who makes the most money, it's the one who makes each man feel special and studly and like she's really, really glad he came.

★ Show that you love what you do—that's why you decided to go pro, isn't it? If you truly want to be there and look forward to seeing people

CAM SITES

Flirt4Free.com

One of the biggest cam sites, with performers. These folks do a great job of marketing and branding the site, and even have a TV commercial.

IMLive.com

Not just for adult performers, this site brings people in with "live experts" in other topics as well. The Sinulator teledildonics system works with this service as well, enabling performers a more intimate level of interaction with fans—and a chance to charge higher fees for the experience.

CamZ.com

Audience members join for free and can chat with performers in the preview area, but must pay to attend your private shows. Women who already have active cam sites of their own get a higher percentage of the take than women who start their performance career at CamZ.

again, they will feel your genuine pleasure and want to come back. Alyssah says her fans can tell she enjoys her work immensely, and that it makes them feel respected and welcomed—because she does respect and welcome them.

★ Creativity is key. If people want to watch porn, they can put in a movie, which is cheaper and easier than spending time at a cam site. Different settings, themes, outfits, and attitudes all go a long way to keeping your work fresh and your fans involved. And you won't get bored either!

★ Seek out women to mentor you. Alyssah recruits women for Flirt4Free, and they work under her, meaning she gets a commission from their earnings. In return, she coaches them on relating to fans, handling the occasional creepy situation, managing their businesses, bringing out their unique erotic personalities, and helping them have a great time with it all. The result? Everyone has more fun, the performers earn more money, and the fans feel like their time and money have been well spent.

How to Become
Internet Famous

HOTTER!

Internet fame is fleeting and fun, and if you live to express yourself, you have no surer road to celebrity. Online, fame and infamy are almost synonymous, especially when it comes to sex. And the best part is, we can all be famous; the roles of star and fan are fluid and ever-changing, so you can flow from one to the other and back again. It's much more fun and egalitarian than Hollywood fame.

If you do set out to become Internet famous with anything having to do with sex or sexual expression, note that it can hurt you if your boss, partner, or family decides to oppose you rather than support your hard work and dedication to creativity.

As with all things Internet—and all things sex, really—you have several routes to choose from. Here are a few to consider.

BLOGGER

More than one sex blogger has landed a book deal after editors noticed her work. Generally, these bloggers had superb writing skills, the ability to create and build a dedicated following, and something unique to say. If you're a good writer and storyteller, blogging might appeal to you—but note that no pseudonym can protect your identity. By all means, use one to create a "brand." Just don't expect it to hide you from employers and family if they go looking.

PERFORMANCE ARTIST

A video camera, broadband, and an exhibitionist streak—along with a talent for stage design—and you can transform your spare room into a burlesque stage, an interpretive sensual dance studio, or a porn set. The key to success is to build your community so that people feel they have a relationship with you and with each other and can incorporate your work into their regular routines. If you're loving it and finding yourself growing in popularity, you might consider going pro and earning some income on the side, if your day job—or your partner— isn't going to dump you if they find out.

WRITER

You don't have to be a full-time writer to have success publishing your erotic fiction. You might not have worldwide recognition, but if your stuff is good, you'll soon be known in the erotica community. And what's generic worldwide fame compared to smaller but more significant esteem from others who are knowledgeable in your field?

VIRTUAL WORLD BUILDER

Any 3D platform that attracts people who want to engage sexually—which, last I checked, is all of them—needs people who can design and build virtual items that facilitate that sex. If you can design or code or market, but not all three, you can partner with people who have the other skills. Second Life residents make actual money from their virtual creations, so along with fame, you can even start to generate . . . well, "wealth" is probably an exaggeration. For now.

ARTIST

From erotic photography to pornographic machinima (movies made in virtual worlds using avatars instead of actors), the Internet community is very supportive of its talented artists. A show of modesty is important in this category, and yet anything digital and visual easily translates between environments. You can have a website, a 3D showcase, and a MySpace profile, all showcasing different aspects of your work.

COMMUNITY LEADER

If you're good at introducing people and facilitating networking and relationship-building, you're the ideal candidate for community leadership. Chat rooms, message boards, special interest groups, remote teams—every community depends on leaders to keep things civil and above board. A community leader may or may not also be the owner or moderator of the group, responsible for banning spammers and approving new members. But community leaders *are* there to mediate disputes, connect people who should know each other, and foster intelligent discussion about the topic at hand. Community leaders automatically take their turn in the spotlight as the group evolves.

VIDEOGRAPHER

YouTube contributors may be the butt of many a joke, but there's no denying that some of that content is at least as good as the professional stuff, and sometimes even better. If you've always wanted to pursue filmmaking as a hobby, this is the time to get started. The audience wants sensual, erotic content that skates that

WHAT SEPARATES THE INTERNET FAMOUS FROM THE INTERNET OBSCURE?

★ A friendly, welcoming attitude that encourages visitors to come back and become part of your community

★ Talent

★ Willingness to share, linking out to others and never dissing the competition

★ Skill at building relationships and communities, and open participation with the audience

★ Media exposure

★ Fresh ideas

★ Good timing, lots of energy, and luck

line of what's allowed on a maintream site like YouTube—which gives you an opportunity to express your sexual imagination without crossing the line into porn. Not that there's anything wrong with that. If that's your beat, check out pornotube.com or xtube.com—but keep in mind that the United States keeps tightening its regulations about recordkeeping and proof that everyone in the film is of age. Search on and read 18 U.S.C. 2257 for the full story before you start publishing pornographic video willy-nilly.

How to Create an Avatar That Looks Like You Feel Inside

 HOT!

I'm one of those people who likes all their digital representations to look as much like their bodies as possible. I want to see *myself* in my electronic image—my avatar—rather than some tall, slender, leggy fantasy self who would probably just make me depressed if I had to watch her too much.

And yet I don't have any design skills. I know what I want but haven't a clue how to manifest it, and frankly, I have no interest in acquiring those skills. That's not the reason I play in virtual worlds, and I'd much rather spend my precious time interacting with people than refining my digital doll.

However.

After a year of being teased by my friends in Second Life for having a blob avatar instead of something custom and cool, I finally took the plunge and went in search of a consultant who could turn me from an egg yolk into a swan. I found two. Duchess Voom and Psyche Etoile showed me how to shop for a "skin" that would provide color and shading and smooth outlines to my shape. They found me a better basic shape to put it on, helped me choose a flattering hairstyle, and taught me how to turn off the built-in animations that

"People really notice when you change your shape and skin around a lot—it makes you look rather schizophrenic. Invest in a good everyday skin. But play with your hair! When I'm feeling sexy, I let my hair down. And if I just feel like having fun, I have pigtails."

—Psyche Etoile, Second Life avatar consultant

keep the avatars moving even when they're standing still. (If I look at it too long, I get seasick.)

Three hours later, my avatar was still short and plump, green-eyed, and freckle faced, just like me. But my edges were smooth, and my face could make expressions, and I no longer shamed my friends when they were seen with me.

Whenever I am faced with creating a visual to represent me, I try to express the way I feel inside in addition to matching my basic dimensions and coloring. I like to be sexy in a rumpled, natural way, to have two-toned hair, and to go barefoot (which has the added bonus of saving me money on shoes). Even the Mii I created to play on my friend's Wii is almost recognizable as *moi,* with her cat glasses and big green eyes.

If you are a designer, animator, 3D modeler—or if you want to be—you probably don't need the tips in this lesson. In fact, you might want to set up shop inside one of the 3D metaverses and sell your skills to n00bs like me who would never be able to deblob themselves.

For the rest of us, here are some pointers.

★ As you have probably gathered, I highly recommend finding an expert—a friend or a consultant whom you pay—to help you create yourself. Think of it as an investment in your future; it saves you time and frees you up to pursue other activities, like cybersex.

★ Ask friends to describe your new avatar to you. I was surprised to find that to most people in Second Life, my porcelain complexion seems to appear zombie white, waxy, and freaky. On my monitor, it's a perfect china doll with shading in all the right places and the cutest sprinkling of freckles where you least expect it. I'm considering choosing a new skin color even as I write this so that my friends and lovers don't have to don sunglasses to play with me in-world.

★ If you want to look like yourself, stick with the basics: hair color, glasses if you wear them, height, general shape. Think of how a police report would describe you, and start there. The more experienced you get with avatars, the more you realize that it really doesn't take much to create a resemblance within the limitations of that particular environment.

★ Meet as many people as you can, so when you see something you like, such as clothing or shoes or hairstyles, you can ask them where they got it.

★ Collect different styles and colors for your hair, so you can have a new style once in a while to change things up, just like you do in real life. Same goes for clothing, accessories, eye color—even body shapes and skin tones.

How to Create a
Pro-Am Webcam Studio

HOTTEST!

Whether you want to become a professional webcam erotic performer or just create a richer sensual experience for a select few of your closest friends, it never hurts to invest in a "professional amateur" home studio. It doesn't matter how great you look on webcam or how brilliant you are at engaging with your lover or audience if they can barely see you due to poor lighting or a blurry picture!

★ Create a personal visual style for your webcam "set." This helps you create mood and atmosphere—not just for you, but for your audience. You might keep several different backdrops around so that you can change the setting as your mood changes. For example, floaty fabrics set a different expectation than leather and chrome.

★ Many digital video camcorders can connect directly to the computer. These units provide higher quality images and audio than a standard webcam. They also "see" better in low light, which lets you get more creative with your lighting.

★ Japanese paper lanterns cast a becoming, diffused light. Or simulate daylight with clip-on lamps from the local home improvement warehouse and blue light bulbs. A small halogen desk lamp, set low and behind your bed or desk, can be an inexpensive backlight that helps separate your body from the background.

★ Remote controls are your friend! You want to be able to adjust the zoom without interrupting the moment.

★ Audio is important for the full sensual experience, and chances are, your camera's built-in mic just isn't strong enough to capture every nuance. Invest in an external microphone that can pick up the full range of sound, from breathing and moaning to slapping and squishing. You'll also have more flexibility in where you position the microphone.

★ Mount your camera on a tripod that you can adjust to various heights. Sometimes you'll want to be on the bed; sometimes you're going to get down on the floor. If you're feeling really fancy and have money to burn, look into a motorized tripod that lets you pan with a remote control.

Part IV:

Just Looking

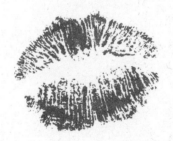

Most of us begin our sex-tech explorations by observing, with or without the intention of getting involved.

"Want to chat?" someone asks. "Just looking," we answer, if we respond at all.

Seeing what the new world of sex has to offer helps us stretch past our own limitations, inspiring us to try something (or someone!) we otherwise would not have thought of, or that used to scare us. Think of it as scouting the territory—or window-shopping, with no pressure to buy.

We want to know what other women are doing, where they're doing it, and why they like it. We read reviews of sex toys, sift through erotica sites for well-written stories, and get bored very quickly with 98 percent of the available pornography.

We lurk in video chat rooms and watch other folks take their clothes off. We go online to play a few rounds of Sudoku and find ourselves more interested in the text chat scrolling by than the game itself. We read about all the crazy sex people are having in virtual worlds like Second Life and wonder how on earth that could be so popular. We know people who say that online dating saved their lives and others who say that all the men on dating sites are creeps—who's telling the truth?

This section contains lessons for anyone who just wants to dip her toe in and test the waters, anyone who is willing to smile at strangers in the crowd but not interested in chatting them up.

Yet.

How to Be a Voyeur
(Without Being a Creep)

 HOT!

You won't need a trench coat and binoculars for this lesson, unless dressing up like a Peeping Tom turns you on—in which case, I'm all for it.

One of the best ways to find out whether something turns you on is to watch other people do it and see how you feel. The Internet has given women the same opportunities to "just look" that men have had for centuries. Now that we know what's out there, we're taking great strides in improving it.

Women tend to prefer interaction, which is one of the reasons many of us enjoy flirting and cybersex more than passively watching porn by ourselves. Voyeurism offers a middle ground, where your participation contributes to the sexual experience of the principals, even though they may not know that you, specifically, are there.

Visit any adult webcam room, and you quickly realize that the exhibitionists in the group need the voyeurs in order to fulfill their fantasies and get the most out of their experience. Just lurking, without a cam of your own, is enough to feed the performers' need for an audience. Your presence fuels their fire, and their uninhibited sexuality can turn you on—and might even inspire you to try something new or exotic with your partner.

ONLINE VOYEURISM CAN:

★ Help you learn new sexual skills

★ Put your own desires into context (you're not alone!)

★ Turn you on

★ Bring you closer to your partner

★ Validate your fantasies

★ Reduce your anxiety

★ Confirm your disinterest

Try chatting with the webcam performer on things not related directly to sex. Unlike DVD performers, these sex workers are not typically professional talent. They're more approachable as regular people. Ask about their day, or the clothes they've chosen, or their love lives. You'll be surprised to find that webcam folks are just like the neighbors.

And if it turns out they are the neighbors? Now you know you have something in common.

Many couples participate in adult communities together, and voyeurism ventures are no different. Watching other people express their sexuality is an ice breaker like no other and can be the catalyst for revealing conversations about sex and its role in your relationship.

How to Lurk in an Adult Chat Room

 HOT!

"Lurking" is the practice of watching a chat without actually chatting. It's a way to get to know the community and figure out whether the group has something to offer you before you commit yourself to an introduction.

It's also a way to get used to the fluid nature of chat. If you've never chatted with multiple people before, the initial immersion can be overwhelming—all those lines of text flowing up the screen! Lurking gives you time to practice sifting the conversations from the noise, to see how people introduce themselves, and to learn some of the acronyms and emoticons in context.

Sounds obvious, right? But there are some tricks to lurking.

★ Read and obey all rules for lurkers and anonymous users. Every chat is different, and the host will have rules that help keep order.

★ Look for an Away or Status setting you can use to help discourage others from private messaging you. Sometimes this status will reset to Available if you click in the chat box, so take care where you click. This is one way to lurk in a 3D virtual world as well.

★ In a webcam room, you can log in without turning on your cam. Or you can put something in front of the camera, like a sign that says AFK (away from keyboard).

★ Chat rooms may have moderators. These people are key members who work to shape the room's interaction. Read the moderator's text to get a feeling for the chat's atmosphere. If you like the moderator's style, you'll likely find the chat room enjoyable.

★ Some webcam chat rooms allow users to log in as a guest. This is like a "designated lurker" label. Guests don't always have all the same room privileges as regular members.

★ Use a different handle every time you log in so that people don't start to recognize your name. You can also use a nondescript, nonfemale name, like "0014," rather than something memorable, like "VenusLovesYou."

★ Ignore all "whispers," private messages, and public posts addressed to your handle and the like. It's not rude to lurk.

★ Keep a shorthand dictionary handy (also known as a chat acronym list) so you can look up things like "rotflmaotntpmp" (rolling on the floor laughing my ass off trying not to pee my pants) and "brb" (be right back) as needed. NetLingo (http://netlingo.com) has a nice starter list.

★ Many residents of 3D worlds keep extra avatars and accounts handy—called alts—for dipping into new clubs, regions, and relationships.

How to Find Porn That Actually Turns You On

HOTTER!

The secret is out: Women are as visual as men, and they like—and watch—pornography. That doesn't mean they like the majority of the product the adult entertainment industry churns out, month after month, for the average male consumer. If you've always thought that porn didn't do anything for you, it probably has more to do with the porn that's easiest to find rather than porn itself.

It's easier than ever for women to find content that turns them on, whether for watching alone or with our partners. And for the first time in history, women have the same access to smut that men have always taken for granted.

One of the great things about online porn is that everybody is represented. The popularity of amateur porn proves that anyone, anywhere, can be a porn star, and that the cliché watermelon-boobs-on-a-toothpick look is not the only option. Even mainstream studios that churn out "professional" product (whatever that means) have niche offerings. Search for "BBW" (big beautiful woman) or "chubby" to see large, voluptuous beauties; "Alt" to see a celebration of body art; "barely legal" for slender hips and smaller breasts; "MILF" for women in their 30s; and "mature" for women 40 and older. (The terms may be offensive, but this is not an industry known for its sensitivity.)

REVIEWER REVUE

Trust the experts to help you find exactly what you're looking for.

Jane's Guide

One of the oldest and best adult review sites can be found at http://janesguide. com. This team of expert reviewers has a lot of experience, as well as a decade of archives, to help you find what you want.

Good Vibrations

Not only does Good Vibes shoot its own videos, it rates all kinds of videos according to a number of important categories: chemistry, plot, production value, natural bodies, good for couples, etc. You can find the ratings on the website (www.goodvibes.com) and in the catalog.

Many women love gay porn because of the focus on raw male sexuality and the beauty of the actors. Most of it seems to be of the wham-bam-thank-you-man variety, although I have seen a few requests from consumers to expand the genre to include more relationship-focused content as well.

One of the fun ways to watch porn is to find an adult community that streams porn as part of the experience. You can find this in webcam rooms and in 3D worlds. Now you have a nice combination of video to watch and people to talk to, all at the same time.

Porn is such a matter of personal taste that it's hard to make specific recommendations, but here are some of my favorite resources to get you started.

MoSex Index

The "taste index" from the Museum of Sex (http://mosexindex.com) takes the collective wisdom of a social network to produce recommendations for each other.

The Smart Girl's Guide to Porn

Violet Blue's book is one of the first to take women's porn interests seriously. Written for the absolute beginner, it's also a useful handbook for those who have experimented quite a bit with porn but haven't found much to satisfy them.

Adult DVD Talk

This video-porn shopping guide website (www.adultdvdtalk.com) contains reviews of DVDs written by volunteer consumer reviewers. It also hosts an online community.

KINK.COM

This family of websites shows authentic, highly erotic sex in various "kinks." Kink.com respects its talent and its audience, and it shows. Start here if you are interested in bondage, dominance and submission, slave training, sex machines, and other forms of alternative sexuality.

PLAYGIRL TV/DVDS

Several of the Playgirl offerings impressed me with the attractiveness of the couples, the quality production values, and the way they focus on the beauty of the male body. It is not "dumbed down" for women, but it is more sensual than standard male-oriented porn. If you're into extreme hardcore, it might bore you. See www.playgirltv.com.

COMSTOCK FILMS

Tony and Peggy Comstock make documentary-style erotic videos starring real-life couples. Shot entirely on film, not video, the Comstocks combine interviews and lovemaking to show each couple in the context of their relationship, not just a random sex scene. See http://comstockfilms.com.

PORNOTOPIA.COM

Sagémonn and Karynna create lovely animated porn with fantasy and science fiction themes. It's not quite Pixar quality, but I find it highly erotic and inspiring, without the gross-out overtones of Japanese-style cartoon porn (a.k.a. hentai).

FOR THE GIRLS

This woman-run porn site for is designed for women and has articles and advice columns, as well as photo and video galleries. See http://forthegirls.com.

FEMALE DIRECTORS

Look for videos from Tristan Taormino, Femme Productions, Nina Hartley, Stormy Daniels, and other female directors to find work that doesn't dismiss women's pleasure out of hand. Independent producers like Audacia Ray and Jamye Waxman are also on the rise.

How to Meet Flirt Buddies While Doing Something Else

 HOT!

Dating sites and adult communities aren't the only place to form relationships online. Many women end up making friends almost without meaning to, in the most casual of situations. For example, the popular games site Pogo.com offers chat rooms alongside many of its card, casino, and puzzle games so players can banter while they play.

As you get to know the other players over time, you end up exchanging IM handles or email addresses and start talking outside of the group. As the months go by, you find yourself incorporating these new friends into your life like any other friend, whether you know them offline or not.

The games engage your mind and give you something to do when the chat room is dull. They also act as a natural filter: Everyone in the chat is interested in the game, so you have something in common to talk about. The games are also tremendously popular. The Entertainment Software Association found that 50 percent of online game play is in this so-called "casual" game space, and that 48 percent of online gamers are women.

OOPS, NOW WE'RE BUDDIES

Places where you can make flirt buddies "on the side," as an adjunct to another activity:

★ Message boards and blogs where you regularly participate in the discussion

★ Shared creative projects like Yelp and Wikipedia

★ Casual game sites like Pogo.com and Yahoo Games

★ Technical support forums and product user groups

★ Live music performances in virtual worlds

Meeting people in a community with a goal—whether it's a game, a fundraiser for a nonprofit, or a music performance—gives you some insight into their character and interests. You can see how people respond when they are winning and losing, whether they are collaborative or competitive or both, and how they treat other people in a nonsexual, nonromantic context.

One caveat: Accidentally finding mates while participating in a common activity is a longstanding human tradition, so be careful not to fool yourself or retreat into denial if you start to form stronger attachments than you think you should.

How to Get Started
in Virtual Worlds

HOTTER!

Virtual worlds, 3D environments, metaverses—whatever you want to call them, this next-generation Internet platform is really just a big dollhouse made electronic so boys could play with it without any threat to their masculinity—even when they want their dolls to be girls.

As a writer and reader, I've always loved the interplay of textual intercourse. I resisted going 3D for a long time because the graphics, animation, and sound were too distracting. But my curiosity got the better of me, and finally, I spent enough time in various 3D environments to get used to the rich media. And now text-only chat seems awfully quiet to me, like I've been cut off from the real activity and locked in a soundproof grey box.

"Once people get used to the immersive environment of 3D, they can't go back to text," says Brian Shuster, CEO of world-building company Utherverse. He's right. When you get through that initial period of discomfort where you keep walking your avatar into walls and you don't know how to find the cool people and your Internet connection isn't quite fast enough to keep up with your controls . . . the rich virtual environment of sound, visuals, and text becomes a natural extension of the rest of your life.

WHAT TO DO FIRST

✔ 1. Pick a world and download the required software.

✔ 2. Register and create your handle. Most worlds allow a free trial period or a free account, which grants you limited access to features.

✔ 3. Read the getting started guide, if there is one, to learn the basics of getting around in-world, customizing your avatar, and pursuing your goals. Also look around the world for designated mentors. Usually these are volunteers who enjoy helping newbies get acclimated.

✔ 4. Customize your avatar. You can generally start playing with a generic, basic avatar, but this marks you as a n00b—a novice, a naïf—and you won't get the full-on experience if you leave it at that.

Entire books have already been written about Second Life, the most famous virtual world as of this writing. That is, famous in mainstream circles. Talk to gamers and veterans of MUDs (Multi-User Dungeon, Domain, or Dimension), MOOs (MUD object-oriented), and any other role-playing game, and they will list a number of other titles before they get to Second Life.

We're not quite at the level of the *Star Trek* holodeck yet, nor have we re-created the *Matrix* as far as I know. But we do have many, many options available when it comes to 3D cyberspace. Instead of trying to list every world, though, I'll give you an overview of the two main camps.

✔ 5. Find a volunteer to show you around, if possible. The designers of Jewel of Indra, a 3D adults-only environment, deliberately designed the world to be difficult to explore on your own. They wanted the community to welcome new members and offer them personal tours of all seven layers of the world. This fosters friendships and community bonds in addition to giving the new person confidence and context at each corner of the tour.

✔ 6. Be patient with technical difficulties. All of these worlds are on the leading edge of technology and suffer from server overload, software bugs, and even—gasp!—the occasional human error.

✔ 7. Talk with people, go to clubs, play the games . . . and when it's time to learn how to use the sex animations, you can always hire an escort to teach you the ropes.

ROLE-PLAYING GAMES

These are the Internet equivalent of running around the neighborhood, protecting the ignorant adults from menaces only children can sense, like aliens, orcs, or monsters. Players sign up and go about normal game business, like collecting objects, fighting enemies, and interacting with other players through their characters. Also known as MMORPGs (massively multiplayer online role-playing games), MUDs, and MOOs, these games ostensibly don't exist to foster romantic relationships, and yet romance and sex abound. You simply can't bring creative, imaginative people into an environment that only exists because all participants agree to contribute to its story and expect them not to liaise. Examples of popular role-playing games include *World of Warcraft* and *The Sims Online*.

3D PLATFORMS

These worlds emphatically point out that they are *not* games. They usually have games in them. But they aren't games in themselves, in the way we think of games. Second Life and Red Light Center are two well-populated examples. Several other platforms are on the horizon.

How to Evaluate a Chat Room in Ten Minutes or Less

 HOT!

It only takes a few minutes to assess a new chat community to see if it's worth sticking around. These tips work whether the community is text-only, webcam, or 3D.

★ Most webcam communities don't require you to have a camera to be in the rooms, although you'll find that the other chatters are more likely to pay attention to you if you are on camera—even if it's not pointed at you—and not everyone shows their faces.

★ How much of the flirting appeals to you, and how much is lame?

★ Do people greet each other when they arrive and have a hard time leaving when it's time to go, because of all the last-minute goodbyes and well wishes? These are signs of a strong core of old-timers who truly value the chat room and work to make it a nice place to be.

LEAVE IF . . .

★ Half or more of the posts are URLs or read like spam subject lines

★ People are calling each other names

★ Nobody says anything for several minutes

★ You get a number of private messages but no one is talking in the public room

★ When you say "Hello, how is everyone today?" you get no responses

STAY IF . . .

★ People greet you and welcome you

★ When you start talking, people talk back

★ At least one good conversation is taking place

★ People seem to know each other

★ Other women seem to be having a good time

★ How much banter and "lol" is there compared to long drawn out silences? Do people play word games? Trivia? Flirt cleverly and explicitly in the public room? People who use their brains make a chat room a blast. If you don't see any signs of intelligent life, move on.

★ Language that is heavy on chat lingo and slang—where complete sentences and grammar are obviously not valued—probably indicate that the maturity level is not where you want it to be.

★ How the community deals with disruptive users also gives clues to how comfortable you will be here. Mature people ignore trolls—users who deliberately insult others or attempt to get into arguments—and good moderators quickly get rid of spammers. When the rest of the folks remain civil and pleasant, you know you've found a good prospect.

★ Different people have different levels of tolerance or preference for adult content. It doesn't take more than a few glances to decide whether this chat room is more or less explicit than what you're looking for.

★ If you see a small group of people carrying on regular conversation that implies they've known each other a while, you're in luck. That's the core group of "regs" that every chat room needs to survive. People who take the time to bond and form friendships or sexual and romantic ties will police the room to make sure it remains a pleasant place. If these sound like folks you want to introduce yourself to and engage with, you've found your chat room.

How to (Politely) Reject
Offers for Cybersex

 HOT!

It's bound to happen. If you're visiting an adults-only community online—and especially if it's a coed area and you sound female—chances are you will be propositioned for cybersex.

I've heard women complain about how often they get propositioned in virtual spaces, whether it's a 3D world or a text chat room. But I compare it to wearing a pretty dress and high heels. If you've obviously done yourself up all nice, people are going to compliment you on it. Likewise, if you're in a space that is designed to facilitate sex, you have to expect that people will ask you about sex.

You are under no obligation to say yes. You cannot be physically threatened or coerced into sexual activity, and you have a Block or Ignore command if the person disregards your polite rejection and begins to pester you.

Online sex can be as much of a challenge for men as offline sex, especially if you are in a situation where you're looking for extended wordplay and flirting,

SUGGESTIONS:

★ "I appreciate your invitation, although I must decline it."

★ "No thank you! But good luck finding what you seek."

★ "Thank you. Maybe another time?" (Caution: Use this only if you are interested in talking with the person in the future.)

★ "No thanks. I am just here to chat tonight."

★ "I'm flattered at your interest, but I am not here for cybersex."

★ "Thanks hon, I'm waiting for my date tho. Good luck!"

and not just a romp on the animated or imaginary sex bed. If he waits too long to make his move, an interested man can end up watching you go off with someone else. If he asks too soon, he can be rejected because you're not warmed up yet.

Very few people have learned how to approach every individual woman in exactly the right way for her. This is no reason to be offended, surprised, or huffy. It's simply part of the landscape. Even if you feel like screaming "Get away from me, you asshole!" you will enjoy yourself more—and so will those around you—if you don't sink to that level.

Online, a polite rejection is more than just good manners. It keeps the vibe pleasant for everyone within text-shot, it keeps you from getting wound up in arguments instead of flirting and playing, and it shows other interested parties the type of approach that doesn't work for you.

When you are consistently respectful and polite, you earn respect and develop relationships that are far more beneficial than the momentary satisfaction of verbally smacking the rude or clueless.

Besides, once you get used to respectfully turning down invitations, you'll feel more comfortable doing the same thing in your offline life. But one tip: If you say no, mean no. Don't start with no and let them wear you down to a yes. That just teaches them to ignore the no and to assume that no eventually means yes. And then the rest of us have a hell of a time fending them off. If you mean maybe, say so!

Part V:

Love

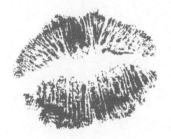

No matter how long you've known someone, you learn more about them and see entirely new aspects of their creativity, their emotions, and their sense of humor when you begin communicating with them through all the various methods modern technology provides.

Writing especially brings out sides of us we don't see at any other time. I've seen this with friends and family as well as with lovers—as soon as we started instant messaging, a new facet of their sense of humor would emerge. One suitor who was too shy to speak words of love was perfectly comfortable writing them, which then led to his being able to say them in person without stuttering.

Combine this wonderful new realm of discovery with the advantage of knowing your partner's body as well as you do, and, well, who knows what could happen?

This section contains lessons for women in committed, ongoing relationships—not necessarily monogamous relationships, but those lovers with whom they have formed lasting bonds. Most of the lessons apply to singles as well, just like almost everything else in this book applies to couples. But this section highlights several ways in which technology can provide new pleasures to long-time partners.

But there's another answer: "Anything you can do with a stranger or a friend, you can do with your partner."

How Not to Fall
in Love Online

HOT!

Ella Fitzgerald: *Louis, Louis, put down that horn a minute. I want to ask you a question.*

Louis Armstrong: *What's on that pretty little mind of yours, there?*

Ella Fitzgerald: *Have you ever been in love?*

Louis Armstrong: *Ain't you solemn! I been in love four times.*

If you've ever been in love, you know that there are as many ways to fall in love as there are people. You might also know that love can sneak up on you when you least expect it, and often when you're actively Not Looking for it.

Falling in love in modern times transcends boundaries: time, distance, technology. Lovers who meet online tend to find ways to shift their schedules to permit frequent interaction, figure out the cheapest ways to travel in order to spend time together in person, and make use of every bit of technology mentioned in this book.

Long-distance lovers finagle joint cell phone plans with unlimited in-plan voice minutes and large packages of text and picture messaging. Better webcams and faster Internet service become priorities, as does your frequent flyer plan and ways to get instant messages through the firewall at work.

Sometimes you have to go through all the work of an active search for True Love before you can honestly set your quest aside and pursue other interests. Love will blossom in its own time (which is usually the least convenient time for you, once you're engaged in your own thing!).

And still other times, we completely screw ourselves up. For every true love that blooms anew online, you'll find the dead petals of a dozen broken hearts. I believe that we need to go through those experiences to mature and appreciate a real love—yet at the same time, if I can save you some steps, I'll gladly do so.

Here are some ways *not* to fall in love online.

★ Have rigid expectations bordering on a checklist for everything you require in a partner.

★ Get involved with multiple partners but demand that each one be exclusive to you.

★ Demand that an online partner be monogamous with you, even though you're in an offline relationship.

★ Rush the relationship. This is easy to do, given that online relationships tend to start from the inside and progress outward. You tell each other the most intimate secrets you hold long before you get to the part about your favorite color. That level of connection makes it feel more natural to leap to Decisions About The Future way too soon.

★ Lie about who you are, what you're interested in, or what matters to you. It's one thing to explore fantasies you wouldn't try offline, or to play different genders or orientations. It's another to lead a partner into a love relationship based on your persona rather than your person.

★ Get so swept up in the drama that you completely lose your common sense. But remember that your body still needs food, water, exercise, and sleep.

★ Fool yourself into thinking you can separate online life from offline life. What happens online doesn't stay online—even if you never meet with the person offline, your emotions are not confined to the Internet.

★ Mistake intensity for love. Online relationships are very powerful because you can interact whenever you're at a computer or using your wireless mobile device. You can quickly build up a codependence that seems like love when it's really mostly habit.

How to Use Technology to Give You More Time for Sex

HOTTER!

We often hope that technology will help us do things faster, better, and with less effort. I'm not sure we always think to prioritize what we'll do with the time we save. And I suspect for most women, the answer is "other work."

It doesn't have to be that way. No errand is more important than your lover (if it is, it's time to rethink the relationship). No completed household task is going to make you as happy as passionate necking on the sofa. Build in more time for sex, and all kinds of good things blossom: glowing skin, relaxed attitudes, more patience with each other, managed blood pressure, physical fitness—the list goes on.

Even something as simple as coordinating your errands to make sure all the household needs are filled and no one needs to make an extra trip to the store frees up time for more romantic pursuits. You can stay on the phone while you hit the grocery store and your partner picks up the dry cleaning, rents a video, and drops the kids off at grandma's. That way, if one of you forgets something, the other can offer a reminder before you're back home and it's too late. Time saved for sex: at least one hour.

Get a robot vacuum and a robot mop to handle the daily mess, and search Craigslist for a housekeeper to come every other week to do the deep cleaning. Time saved for sex: 15–45 minutes a day.

Use a shared online calendar to plan surprises for each other. Create appointments like "Tuesday, 8:00 PM, oral sex in the shower" and follow up on the promises. (Make sure you set the calendar to "private" and give only you and your partner access to it, unless you want to show your sex schedule to the whole world.) Google's calendar works well for this purpose. Time saved for sex: however much time you schedule and use.

Use a personal video recorder like TiVo to capture the television you want to watch and have sex earlier in the evening. You can always watch TV after sex, whereas if you watch TV first, sometimes you're too tired for lovemaking afterwards. And if you end up drifting off to sleep in a postcoital cocoon of love and devotion, you can always rent the DVDs later. Time saved for sex: an hour for dramas, or 30 minutes for sitcoms.

Sign up for fare alerts and last-minute travel deals at your favorite airlines and travel websites. Then mark a few dates on your shared online calendar to keep them available for a romantic getaway. Email everyone on your "support team"—babysitter, pet sitter, housesitter, etc.—and have them plan to take care of things for those days. You won't know where you're going until the last minute but you sure know what to do once you get there! Time saved for sex: hours of advance planning, plus 2–5 days of getaway time.

Sign up for regular grocery or meal delivery services so you can spend less time prepping meals and more time enjoying each other. Every city has its own set of local services, or you can look into a larger operation like *DineWise* (www.

dinewise.com) or Schwans (www.schwans.com), which serve several major American cities and some smaller towns too. Google "meal delivery service" + your town to find local options ranging from organic produce delivery to full dinners from local restaurants. Time saved for sex: Up to an hour a day, depending on how often you get things delivered.

If you have a regular paycheck and sign up for automatic deposit, sign up for automatic bill pay as well. Get cash back when you shop so you never have to go to the bank or sit at the table and pay a month's worth of bills. Time saved for sex: an hour a month.

How to Make Love a Game

HOTTEST!

Sex games for couples have come a long way from the flashcards of yesteryear, but some still follow the classic form of giving you an action to perform with your lover. The advantage of going digital is that you have almost endless possibilities, thanks to expansion packs and the ability to customize the text and add new activities on the fly.

Bliss is a sex game that takes a bit of Cranium, a bit of Monopoly and a whole lot of Kama Sutra and stirs them together into a different-every-time-you-play erotic experience for couples.

Creators Don and Suzanne, who have been married to each other for twenty-five years, developed Bliss with one overall goal: to help couples stay together. "Everyone wants a relationship to last, and sometimes it seems too hard in this world," says Suzanne. "But there's no reason it can't get better and better."

Game play is simple. Click to roll the dice, and watch your game piece move the designated number of spaces on the (virtual) board.

Each space represents "land" that you can buy and develop; instead of Monopoly-style hotels and houses, you build massage parlors, strip clubs, art studios, and the like. When your piece stops, the game presents you with instructions about what to do while you're in that space.

And that's where it gets interesting. Because unlike an old-fashioned erotic board-and-card game, basic Bliss starts with five hundred "actions" for couples to perform.

These actions are smart too.

Every time you start the game, you complete an "available toys" inventory, listing everything you have handy. This can range from ice cubes, bed sheets, and flavored lubes to vibrators, ballpoint pens, and cameras.

The game then knows what you have around to play with. As I discovered, the more you have handy, the more fun the game becomes. (You might be surprised at how many common household objects become erotic, given the right context.)

The next step is a clothing checklist. Don spent a lot of time developing a complex algorithm that not only tracks what you've taken off or put back on, but also considers the relationships between garments.

"Bliss knows you can take off a baby doll if you're wearing pants, but you can't take off a teddy without undoing your pants," he says. And the game shouldn't ask you to take off any attire you're not currently wearing.

Finally, each player sets his or her starting "passion level" on a scale of one to nine. This ensures you're not expected to go down on your partner when you're still thinking about the presentation you're giving on Tuesday. It also balances things out if one of you is hornier than the other.

For example, when I started at passion level two ("Cold"), the game assigned my partner the action of looking in my eyes and telling me why he thinks I'm wonderful. For 30 seconds. (I told you this was a good game!)

But because he started at a four ("Warm"), the game assigned me more provocative activities to do for him. Eventually we noticed that our passion meters had synched up and that our assigned actions involved similar levels of effort.

You can adjust your personal profile to reflect your tastes, including assigning various sexual activities to certain passion levels. You won't be assigned an action until you've reached its associated passion level.

"I've had customers who see oral sex as not much different from kissing," Don says. "Others see it as more intimate than intercourse."

Matching actions to passion levels becomes even more important when you add expansion packs, which add kinkier actions and incorporate creative assignments requested by customers. You set your preferences to keep what you like and exclude what you don't, so you aren't given an action halfway through the game that completely wrecks your mood.

Permission, says Suzanne, is a big part of the game. You might secretly want to dim the lights, put on a special song, and strip for your lover, and yet you might be shy about mentioning it. But if the game tells you to do it, well, you have to do it.

"Bliss removes all the blocks," Suzanne says. "You get to say what you want, what you like. And even if you're feeling completely different from each other—one is hot and one is cold—sex isn't out of the picture. Why would it be?"

Naturally, I poked around the game on my own before inviting my playmate to join me. Without telling him, I set my profile to avoid giving me actions in which I had to be highly aggressive or dominant, as I lean toward submissiveness (in sex, anyway).

But after our first game, I went into the action editor to change the text on some of the existing actions. I adapted some of the actions to reflect my personal history, my tattoo, a specific freckle, the color of my sheets, and various other unique elements. That alone is worth the extra cost for the action editor license, even if I never create a new action from scratch.

I also added some of my own MP3s to the music directory. It's easier to get into the actions that require music when you're familiar with the songs.

The action editor is not a sexy interface, and creating your own actions is more complicated than it seems. You have to consider all the variables. Does your action require a player to remove a bra? What if the person's not wearing one?

I recommend fiddling with the action editor at a time other than when you're playing the game together. You can also visit the Action Exchange board on the website (www.gamesforloving.com), where you can swap actions and programming advice with other enthusiasts.

But the action editor is also your key to total personalization, a way to surprise your partner with favorite fantasies, clothing, and props only you two know about.

The game never quite gets to the point of telling you, "Stop playing the game and go finish having sex." Rather, the assignments become more open-ended and vague when your passion meters reach level nine. Instead of "Dance naked for two minutes," you are now instructed to "Improvise" and "Take as long as you need."

How to Make Love to a Nerd

HOTTEST!

While the Internet has long been mainstream and is no longer the secret clubhouse of the geeky set, chances are, if you get into online community and online sex, you're going to be spending time with nerds.

You lucky, lucky girl.

I'm going to hit on the stereotype a bit here; this doesn't hold true for all people who identify as "nerds" or "geeks," but it's common enough that it warrants us taking it seriously.

The classic nerd tends to be shy, interested in science fact and fiction, and inexperienced with girls despite a rich fantasy life. That actually makes the classic nerd brilliant in cyberspace.

★ Don't expect your nerd to know what to do, no matter how enthusiastic he or she is about doing it.

★ Do expect your nerd to have seen online porn. You might want to go look at some yourself, so you know the kinds of things he or she has seen.

ONLINE DATING FOR NERDS

Science Connection
http://sciconnect.com

Geek to Geek
www.gk2gk.com

Sweet on Geeks
http://sweetongeeks.com

Nerd v. Geek
I've always defined "geek" as "nerd + cool," but apparently that's a fairly regional usage centered around the San Francisco Bay Area. For the purpose of this lesson, I use both terms synonymously. Your geek lover may have an entirely different idea about what is geek and what is nerd. A strong opinion on this is one of the signs of geekdom. And nerdiness.

★ Nerds come in many flavors: science, technology, comic books, Star Wars, assorted sci-fi TV shows, role-playing games, Internet, and more. Sex is a lot better when you share the same passion as your nerd.

★ To send your nerd a special sentiment, follow the online comic strip xkcd (http://xkcd.com), which is written by a nerd with a deep understanding of the human heart. You are bound to find something in the archives that speaks to even the most romantic geek.

How to Get Your Lovers to Send You Hot Text Messages, Even If They Don't Want to at First

HOTTER!

It's almost incomprehensible, but did you know that many people aren't interested in hot texting?

Shocking, I know.

But if you are at all word oriented, your lover needs to make an effort to connect with you in this way. No ifs, ands, or buts. It's amazing, what those 160 characters can do. They can say "I'm thinking of you" or "I love you" or "I want to bury myself between your thighs and not come up until you've climaxed six times." Sometimes all that in a single message.

I understand that if your phone doesn't have a comfortable keyboard, a text message can be a laborious missive to craft. I also understand that if you love someone who needs that interaction, you will gladly accept the burden—and learn how to use predictive text to minimize your keystrokes.

These are some of the ways I've had success in teaching lovers to text me.

★ Ask them to text you sometimes, and explain how much you appreciate their effort and thoughtfulness. Remind them it doesn't have to be Nobel Prize–winning poetry, just an honest note.

★ Send them hot texts telling them what you want to do with them next time you see them, and then following through, so they see clearly that hot text is foreplay and leads to great lovemaking.

★ Point out that song lyrics that have meaning for you make wonderful text messages.

★ Include questions in your texts to them from time to time, to encourage response.

★ Make sure not to demand or expect a response every time, so they don't feel pressured—that takes the fun out of it.

★ Show them a way they can text your phone from a web interface. Google and Yahoo both make applications that let you send a message to almost any phone, as do the phone companies.

★ Sign yourselves up for Twitter (http://twitter.com), a microblogging service that helps friends keep in touch by providing a central address to post quick messages about where you are, what you're thinking, and what you're doing. These messages can be sent and received via your mobile device or the web.

★ Remind them that pictures are worth a thousand words, so even if a picture message costs more to send, it's also worth 58 text messages.

★ Outline the benefits of texting over calling. It's more discreet, it can be replied to later, it often works when voice calls fail, and it creates a minilog you can go back and read.

★ Short words work really well in text. Think of all the wonderful four-letter nouns and verbs the two of you can share. Unlike email, there's no big blank page daring you to fill it up.

★ Most phones offer a way to save phrases you want to use often. The dozen or so that come standard with the phone are rarely interesting enough to be worthwhile—but your lovers can add their own as they think of them.

How to Reassure Your Man That Sex Toys Won't Replace Him

HOTTER!

More often than you'd think, men worry about being replaced by sex-oriented technology. They fear that their penises—which cannot vibrate or rotate and do not come with multiple attachments or clitoral stimulators in cute animal shapes—will no longer be enough after a woman gets her first ride on a jumbo-size rabbit pearl.

The analogy I've been using to lay those fears to rest is this: Sex toys are like almonds. Almonds can be a delicious and satiating snack on their own. Almonds can be a delightful addition to a salad, trout, a bowl of cereal, yogurt, or a dessert. You can share almonds with others, or enjoy them on your own.

But few people want to replace every meal with a bowl of almonds for the rest of their lives.

And few people want to replace human touch and intercourse—or love!—with tools, no matter how advanced our technology becomes. You will no more replace your man with toys than he will replace you with porn. Besides, those who prefer inanimate objects to human lovers aren't good candidates for sexual relationships anyway.

Yet it's important to treat his anxieties with respect. Think of how you would feel if he laughed or ignored your groundless worries.

★ Take him to a sex-positive store or website and look at toys together, reading the articles that tell you different ways to use them and focusing on devices intended for couples.

★ Remind him that the more orgasms you have, the more orgasms you want. Using toys with yourself keeps you feeling sexual overall. As one of my friends puts it, "Having fries with my burger doesn't make me not want a burger. It just makes me crave the meal again. And again. Are you busy right now?"

★ If your vibrators leave you too numb to feel his caresses, acquire some other toys for the day before you see him, or take time off from the toys now and then. The Je Joue and the Eroscillator both offer ways to stimulate the clitoris without high-revving vibrations.

★ Ask him why he thinks he could be replaced by an object that cannot tell you jokes, hold you when you need to cry, or warm the bed on a winter night. If he truly fears that he cannot offer your more intimacy and pleasure than a battery operated device . . . why is he in this relationship in the first place?

★ Use the toys with him so he can see how nonthreatening they are, and that they are just part of everyday sexuality. If he's shy, tell him you will be in heaven if you can lie back and let him play you like a violin—and that you will return the favor next time.

How to Shop for Gifts for an Online Lover

HOT!

The Internet makes it easy to send gifts to your lovers, even if you've never exchanged your legal names or mailing addresses.

IF YOU HAVE YOUR LOVER'S EMAIL ADDRESS . . .

★ Peet's Coffee & Tea lets you send an eCup to one or more lovers all at once. Starting at $1.70 for a coffee and $3.75 for an espresso-based drink, it's a thoughtful way to show you care without busting your budget.

★ The iTunes store supports online lovers with the Gift This feature. Songs, albums, movies, TV shows, e-books—if it's digital, you can send it. You can even gift playlists you put together yourself: the modern equivalent of the mix tape.

★ Donations to charities can be made online in others' names, and no one cares whether the name is an IM handle.

IF YOU HAVE YOUR LOVER'S SNAIL MAIL ADDRESS . . .

★ Buy two candles of the same scent and ship one to each of you to burn while you chat.

★ Mail your lover a gift, but leave the familiar territory of Amazon.com for stores that have products likely to hold meaning for online relationships, including ThinkGeek (www.thinkgeek.com), GiftsForEngineers.com and The Tech Museum of Innovation (http://thetech.org) store. If you need some help in knowing how to gift your geek, check http://gizmodo.com and www.engadget.com for ideas.

★ Create sexy digital files—photos, video, audio, erotica—and send them on a USB drive that uses mandatory user passwords. Your lover must follow your clues or instructions to "earn" the right to be told the passwords. Look for secure USB drives that lock out the hacker after ten password failures, in case of theft.

IF YOU HAVE YOUR LOVER'S HOME ADDRESS . . .

★ Have a week's worth of groceries—or perhaps special gourmet items people wouldn't normally splurge on for themselves—delivered right to your lover's door. (Someone will have to be home to sign for it.) This is fun for sending ingredients and then making the same dish or meal together while connected by Skype.

★ Using an online guide to local business like Yelp or Citysearch, find some neat and unexpected service to hire for your lover. Arrange for a mobile dog groomer, send a gardener over to plant a dwarf lemon tree, or treat your lover to an in-home massage.

★ Use an online map tool to create a guide of fun things to do within five miles of your lover's house. Parks, historical buildings, coffee houses—show your lover that he or she doesn't have to go far to get some culture and exercise to get refreshed for your next long online session.

How to Talk to Your
Lover About Porn

HOTTER!

Porn is now easier to find than bras that fit. This forces many women to face up to their feelings about their partner's looking at adult content. Some women feel that their lovers will develop unrealistic expectations about female bodies or athletic ability after watching a lot of porn; others worry that the fantasy that pornography provides will replace the reality of everyday sex.

Yet we know that forbidding something just makes it more desirable. And given the benefits we reap from sexual exploration, I suggest incorporating some pornography into the sexual routine so that everything stays in balance, rather than issuing an ultimatum that your lover has to choose between porn or you.

★ If your lover is a man, porn is probably going to be a part of his sex life. Porn and boys go together like girls and toys. Don't let it scare you. Share it with him, at least to a certain extent. (Everyone needs a little private time sometimes too!)

★ You can learn about each other from the kinds of porn that turn you on—especially if you're shy about revealing what you like, or if you feel tempted to share video that you think you should like but that doesn't actually do much for you.

★ Watching adult videos together can help you transition from being parents and workers to being lovers —it's like taking off the suit and slipping into a bath at the end of a long day.

★ Seeing what turns the other on can make you better sexual partners, both in the sense of trying out what you've seen and in the conversations you have about what turns you on through film that you don't want to try yourself.

★ Keep your mind open. It's not nice to yuk someone's yum. Sex is a very personal thing—and you might be surprised at what turns you or your lover on. Remember that watching it isn't the same as doing it. Even if you lover is into porn themes that turn your stomach, you aren't necessarily expected to act it out, nor are you under any obligation to do so.

How to Understand What You're Getting into Online

HOTTER!

Online relationships tend to follow a similar pattern, regardless of the tools you use: text, audio, video, 3D, mobile. It's one of those things you see clearly in other people but don't always realize you're caught up in it until it's too late—quite possibly wonderfully too late.

This is a typical online relationship arc that I've seen played out hundreds of times in the past dozen years or so. I've been through it more than once myself.

✔ 1. You find a community that appeals to you.

✔ 2. You start getting to know people, bantering and flirting, and returning regularly.

✔ 3. You become more explicit in your flirting and start to home in on one or more potential partners, people who give good word, who take your breath away. People who you look for. You start logging in every night and hanging out well past your bedtime in hopes that they will show up. Then, when they do, you sometimes chat until dawn without even realizing it.

✔ 4. You spend more and more time online with your lover, discovering more about them and marveling at their marvelousness. You are both pouring out your souls and feeling like you are being understood like never before. The intimacy and depth of your connection is profound and life-altering.

✔ 5. You blend this relationship into your life. You give it priority as one of the most important relationships you have and you defend it to those who claim that online relating is fantasy or fake.

✔ 6. You reach a Dramatic Event. At this point, you are deep in the relationship, and the drama has been escalating along with the emotional bond. This is a point of no return: Either you break it off and drift through your life bereft and heartbroken (for a while at least), or you meet in person to see whether your chemistry exists beyond the web, or you agree Once And For All to keep your relationship solely online. The Dramatic Event tends to happen 3–18 months into the relationship, although this varies from person to person. If you already have a partner, the Dramatic Event might be that your online relationship has been discovered or has taken on more significance than your preexisting relationship can bear.

✔ 7. You start to regain your life balance. Between the Dramatic Event and now, you might go through tremendous pain, but that too shall pass. Or maybe you just wake up one day and realize you haven't seen the sun for a year. You might continue to visit the community once or twice a week; some women take several months off entirely. Couples who meet in online communities often stay in touch with their mutual friends. On the flip side, you might have found the exact right balance of online and offline time—or the right balance of each lover if you have more than one—and feel centered and whole in a way you've never felt before.

Your relationship might not follow this pattern, of course. Yet so many people get into trouble by thinking they are exempt from the pitfalls of online involvement, I think it's important to acknowledge the general progression that most of us experience. Denying what you're getting into just makes things that much harder if the relationship goes sour or starts to cause problems in the rest of your life. But if you can accept and even embrace the milestones as they arise in your online relationship you will be prepared to do the work required to keep your life balance, both online and off.

How to Feel Closer When You're Apart

 HOT!

Long-distance or traveling lovers have so many ways to stay in touch these days. This is a not an exhaustive list by any means, but it should be enough to get you started.

SKYPE

More than one couple keeps Skype on all day, whether they're at their computers or not. Skype is free and connects you through voice, text, and webcam. I've kept it on voice all day while we're both working—not talking, just listening to each other breathe.

MICROBLOGGING

Services like Twitter and Jaiku provide a fun way for couples and their friends to keep in touch. It's a simple idea: Through the web, IM, or a cell phone, you send a short message to a central address. This started out as a way to tell your friends where you're going—"@ bill's place, 9:00 PM"—so they could join you. But the community quickly expanded it to include thoughts, quotes, song lyrics, and even have conversations in shorthand. You can have messages sent to your mobile device and feel connected anywhere you have cell service. It's fun to do this with a small group of close friends; otherwise you'll be overwhelmed with messages, and the point here is to feel like even though you're in a long-distance relationship, you have a close group to hang out with.

SHARING THE MUSIC

SimplifyMedia (http://simplifymedia.com) lets you and your lover listen to each other's music libraries over the Internet, even the copyright-protected files, as long as you both log in with the same user name. You can invite up to thirty friends to share libraries, so it works for polyamorous groups as well as couples. At press time, the software was still in beta and worked only with iTunes; support for other players is on the way.

LISTENING TO THE RADIO

Many local radio stations offer Internet streams now, so if one of you is away from home, you can still feel close not just to each other but to your home. Or pick a radio stream or podcast to listen to together. This is especially nice if you're at work and can't be overheard typing into IM windows or muttering into a Skype microphone.

INSTANT MESSAGING

Once you get into the groove, you might be able to IM alongside any other work or school project you've got going. It might seem awkward at first, but for many people (including me), it soon becomes so natural to talk with a lover while working that it becomes harder to work without IM going than with the connection open. I've found that leaving the IM window open makes it easier to go "heads down" and work for a set period of time, half an hour or an hour or so, without posting a new IM—and yet still feel connected to my partner. Some folks find this incredibly distracting and never get into the groove: If that's you, close it, because your long-distance relationship is not well served by getting yourself fired.

BUILDING A VIRTUAL HOME

Second Life, Red Light Center, Jewel of Indra—pick an environment that appeals to you and build yourself a nest. You can decorate it together, stream videos into your virtual TV to watch movies together, or just hang out in bed together while you talk about your day.

How to Break Up
with an Online Lover

 HOT!

It doesn't take long to figure out that relationships are relationships, wherever you develop them. And you know as well as I do that sometimes love relationships need to come to an end.

Breaking up in person is hard enough, but how do you end an online relationship? True, you don't have to watch anyone crumble and weep. But this is someone you have probably shared your deepest soul with—certainly, your sexual fantasies and desires have come up a time or two in conversation. You have chat logs dating back to the beginning, mutual online friends, perhaps even joint property if you're in a game or virtual world.

You could just change all your handles, block him or her in all the tools you use, and never go back to the places you shared. Or you could strap it on and do what needs doing, out of love and respect.

Breakups are as individual as relationships, but these are some general guidelines to help you through this painful time.

★ Use a real-time technology like IM or private chat to break the news, not email.

★ Set aside plenty of time for a conversation to make sure the other person has a chance to have his or her say.

★ If you both hang out in the same community, you might need to try not to be in the room at the same time for a while. If it's a mutual parting of the ways, this might not be a concern.

★ Do your best to keep things civil and respectful. You probably have naked pictures of each other, chat logs you wouldn't want splashed on the front page of the newspaper, and secrets about each other's hopes and dreams. You're not going to post those on the Internet to fulfill some immature revenge fantasy; don't give the other person the inspiration to do so either.

★ Don't put mutual friends in the position of having to report on what the other is doing.

★ Follow the steps in How to Delete Your Ex, page 186, as needed.

How to Delete Your Ex

HOT!

When modern relationships end, they leave behind more artifacts than a pharaoh's tomb. Email, instant messages, text messages, voicemails, digital pictures, and video—and that's just the personal stuff. What about blog posts? Social networks? That tandem skydiving video you posted to YouTube?

You can't do much about artifacts that have already gone public, but you can reduce your chances of stumbling upon a memento unprepared.

★ Block every IM handle your ex gave you and remove them from your buddy lists.

★ Set your IM clients to accept messages only from people already on your buddy list.

> If you're not ready to put your ex away for good, you still might want to place the relics of your relationship into a special . . . well . . . reliquary. In that case, create a folder to move the items into instead of the trash.

MY EX, MYSPACE

You can do a lot to clear your ex out of your hard drives and mobile devices, but how many ways are the two of you connected in the outside world? If you've been together a while, chances are you are linked together on MySpace, LinkedIn, LiveJournal, Twitter, and/or many, many other social networking sites.

Whether you remove or block each other completely depends greatly on how the breakup happened, the residual feelings you have for each other (affection? irritation? restraining order?), and how much time you want to spend visiting every community site where you are connected. Removing each other from your Friends lists can have a ripple effect through your social group as your friends have to figure out whether they are now your friend, your ex's friend, or somewhere in the middle, staying friends with both (or neither) of you.

You might want to leave the networking sites alone for the nonce and see how you feel in three or six months. Unless your ex is harassing you through your profile, it is likely okay just to leave things as they are.

★ Remove your ex from your contact list so you don't make yourself crazy monitoring his or her online habits.

★ Destroy all email, both from and to. Don't forget to search for your ex's address in the "cc" and "bcc" fields, as well as the "to" field.

★ If your ex knows about your online dating profile, see whether you can block him or her from contacting you through it. (Some sites don't have this feature, alas.)

★ Check My Pictures, My Documents, and your attachments folder for images to send to the trash.

★ Delete your ex's email from your address book, including from lists of multiple recipients. Don't forget to check your mobile devices too.

★ Delete your ex's Mii from your Wii. Note that it might reappear in the Mii parade. Keep deleting as needed.

Part VI:

Sex

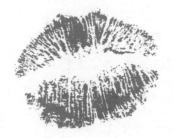

How can you have sex with a computer? You can't.*

But you can have sex with people long-distance if your mental, spiritual, or emotional connection is strong enough. Couples have been doing it for years with whatever technologies are available to them—letters, telegraph, telephones, email, instant message . . . the list goes on. We have so many options for keeping the fires burning, and in fact, some of the modern ways to have long-distance sex require a deeper understanding, trust, and intimacy than physical sex.

Sex online can lead to broken hearts online and broken relationships offline. But it can also be a place of discovery, a place for fun, a place for healing, and a place to build sexual self-esteem. It all depends on your attitude, expectations, and willingness to experience.

If you're single, fling yourself into it like a teenage football player at the buffet. If you're not, be careful, and make sure to discuss boundaries and discoveries with your partner if you want to keep the relationship healthy and alive.

This section covers both online and offline sex, helping you avoid the pitfalls and get right to the pleasure.

---

* Well, you can, but I would argue that's really sex with yourself—which is a noble pursuit in itself, and you can learn more about it in the Self-Discovery section.

How to Puzzle Your Lover

HOTTEST!

Let other couples worry about losing the mystery—you know that puzzles, conundrums, and enigmas keep love fresh. Couples who think together not only give their brains a fun workout, they learn problem-solving skills that serve them well in other areas of the relationship. These tips offer something for everyone: a visual puzzle to create for one another, a bit of friendly competition on the seven seas, and a plethora of casual challenges you can do without getting out of bed or rolling any dice.

JIGSAW

Start with a sexy full-body picture of yourself, either in the nude, in lingerie, or in fetish costume.

Open a copy of the picture in a graphics editor, or use a screen-capture program like SnagIt, and make a number of smaller images, each containing a small part of the original image (a hand, the curve of a thigh, an ear, etc.).

Send one small image to your lover each day.

Have your lover assemble the pieces and send you the final image when it's all finished.

PIRATES

Sign up for Puzzle Pirates (www.puzzlepirates.com), an online role-playing game in which players form crews and sail the high seas in search of booty. As you might imagine from the title, pitched battles do occur—battles of wit and logic, that is. Instead of fighting with cutlass and dagger, these pirates solve puzzles; whoever solves them faster, bigger, and better wins the day. The avatars are cute and round-headed, resembling nothing so much as those little plastic Fisher-Price people, and the only "adult" content in the game is what you and your lover make up in private chat as you go.

But here's a hint: It's even more fun if you play on separate teams, but from the same room in the house.

POGO

Pogo.com is the home of numerous casual games, from poker to word searches to Sudoku. You can play together from anywhere, whether on the same computer or bringing two laptops to bed—or two laptops from anywhere in the world.

Keep it casual with simple play, or spice it up with your private rules. Maybe the winner gets two minutes of whatever they like from the loser; maybe the loser has to lose an article of clothing, or perform a household chore. If you're apart, think up diabolical consequences you can do from afar; send payment in the form of a digital picture of a particular body part or pose, maybe, or perform a dance or striptease via webcam.

When you're together, you can have your partner play a game against strangers or Internet buddies while you indulge in intimate, delicious acts upon their body. Can they still beat the international crowd at checkers while you are licking and suckling the skin behind their knee?

How to Seduce Someone in 160 Characters or Less

HOTTEST!

Text messages are the best thing for couples since the invention of the cell phone. It doesn't matter if you're freshly dating or if you've been together for years—a text is the perfect compromise between flirting and productivity.

Text is the least disruptive way to connect. If you're busy, you can look forward to checking your phone when you have a moment. You can text from anywhere, while standing in line, while waiting at red lights, while on hold with a mortgage lender, in the restroom when you're out to dinner with someone else. You can share that romantic, sexy, or funny thought immediately after it occurs to you. And then you can relax and forget it, because you don't have to store it up to tell each other later.

No one has to know you're doing it. Unlike a phone call, texting is a private activity that you can perform in a public place. That means you can get as mushy or as naughty as you please without annoying (or exciting) those around you. Don't forget to set your phone to vibrate or silent mode so incoming messages don't harsh anyone's mellow.

DIRTY TALK OR CASUAL CONVERSATION?

One friend confessed to me the deliciously dirty texts her boyfriend had been sending her while he was away on business. She giggled as she repeated his latest: "Send me a picture, and get real close. I want to see the pink." Then she paused and blushed a little. I was still waiting for the dirty part, until I realized that for them, that was incredibly daring.

Everyone has a different idea of what is delightfully risqué and what is disturbingly rude. Work within your lover's limits at first, and if that seems acceptable, you might push a little and see if the boundaries can expand. If not, back off. You want texting to be both hot and safe, and it's not the best medium for deep discussions about limits.

THE JOY OF TEXT

While a simple "Come over and do me" text message works on just about anyone, it skips the whole seduction part. Yes, you are seducing . . . but done right, a steamy exchange of texts will beguile a lover as well, if not more.

Honesty is more important than fancy prose. Most paramours would rather receive a genuine "thinking of you" (or "TOY") than have you so frozen from writer's block that you don't text at all.

Texting, like instant messaging, tends to bring out our wilder sides. If you're just getting to know a new flame, keep your tone flirtatious, and let them signal whether they are open to more explicit language. For example, you might send something like "I can still taste your kiss." This is both

TEN TIPS FOR TITILLATING TEXT

★ Mix it up. Be romantic, funny, erotic, matter-of-fact, and pornographic by turns.

★ Use abbreviations sparingly, but use them when you need them.

★ In the beginning of a new hetero relationship, the woman is usually the one to set the tone (for example: family, flirty, or filthy).

★ Sometimes it's hotter to use the longer word rather than the shorter one.

★ Triple-check the recipient's address before you press Send.

★ It's better to craft original text than paste canned phrases from a list. But it's okay to quote song lyrics, books, movies, and anything else that holds meaning for the two of you.

★ Women are often more sexually explicit in text messages than they are out loud. At first.

★ You can send text messages to a lover's phone from the web. Go to the website of their wireless service provider and search for the "Send TXT" link. Enter the recipient's phone number, type your message, and click Send.

★ You know the relationship is going well if the two of you start developing an SMS shorthand all your own.

★ If texting becomes part of the foundation of your relationship, invest in a phone with a QWERTY keyboard.

romantic and erotic, and it can have several shades of meaning, depending on what the two of you have been up to. If the reply includes more detail about which body parts got kissed, you can follow up with juicy descriptions of exactly what you will do next time. But if you get a smiley and "Thanx!" in return, you might want to avoid writing anything that could be published in *Penthouse*.

Song lyrics and movie quotes make excellent personal messages. Simple phrases like "love your chin" or "I was just thinking about how great you look walking around in just a towel" work great too. The important thing is that you mean what you say, when you say it.

Text in regular language. This is romantic: "You are my breath. You are the very heart of me, responsible for every pulse of blood in my veins." This is not: "ur my breth. ur d vry hart of me, responsibl 4evry pulse of bl%d n my veins."

Let the teenagers plague their English teachers with SMS lingo. Write like a grown-up.

If you text enough, you'll find yourself running through mental lists of synonyms, trying to find the shortest word possible that still says what you mean. I have a whole vocabulary of four-letter words to substitute for longer words in text messages. For example, I use "alas" instead of "I'm sorry" and "ergo" instead of "therefore."

Couples often develop their own shorthand. One friend uses "[t]" to stand for "team," which is how she and her partner think of themselves. Another spent a giddy week early in the relationship exchanging every word they could think of that started with L—list, lodge, ludicrous, lurk, lorry, luminous, luscious— until one day, eventually, they worked up to the real thing: love.

Beware the Freudian send. This is when you send a message to the wrong person—typically, the person you least wanted to receive it. You want to be extra, super-duper careful if you are dating more than one person (or having an affair). Sending a generic "You're fantastic!" to the wrong person isn't going to wreck anything. But sending "I loved that thing you did with your tongue last night" to a partner you haven't called for a week is not going to make anyone's day.

How to Show Your Boobies Without Ending Up on YouTube

HOTTEST!

To avoid Internet infamy, you have to show your beautiful naked body only in person and never allow anyone to bring a cell phone—or a PDA, or a security camera, or a spy pen—within range.

But what fun is that? If you want to play with exhibitionism, but worry about becoming the next hot amateur sex tape, follow these guidelines to minimize your risk.

★ Only share revealing photos with people you trust absolutely. If they really love you, they'll delete the files at your request or encrypt their collection. If nothing else, they will keep the pictures on a local drive and never redistribute them on the Internet.

★ Keep your face out of the frame, especially when you're playing in chat rooms. Webcam images are easily captured and republished by unscrupulous chatters.

ANNUAL BLOGGER BOOBIETHON

Every year, the Blogger Boobiethon collects pictures of breasts and uses them to raise money for breast cancer research. The pictures are organized into two galleries—a free section where anyone can few the clothed breasts, and a restricted section, where you have to make a donation and assert that you are of legal age in order to see the bare breasts.

Men and women alike donate their photos, and many get creative with their decorations, painting pink ribbons on their chests, writing the name of a loved one who had breast cancer, or getting a little sexy with bras and lingerie. Women who have had mastectomies proudly display their scars. The photos are tasteful and celebratory, and the event maintains an uplifting spirit.

If you later decide to share those pictures with your lovers (*after* they have made the donation to see them in the gallery, mind you), and the pictures leak, you can always point out to family and employers that you were helping raise money for breast cancer, and that they should be ashamed of themselves for throwing it in your face.

Pictures are collected each year at the end of September, and the event runs from October 1 through October 8.

★ Get artful with draped fabric, scarves, shadows, and large hats and glasses to conceal, even as you reveal.

★ Crop images or pose for photos that only show partial breast. A nipple or a curve or a shadow of cleavage can all be wonderfully erotic and yet aren't as immediately recognizable as you.

★ Computers, iPods, USB sticks—anything a person can store pictures on can be stolen. This happened to a friend of mine, whose hard drive was stolen out of her luggage at an airport. It happened to be the drive she and her boyfriend used to store the digital records of their long-distance relationship, and we all had some tense weeks while we waited for the compromising photos to wind up online. They never did, and most likely, the thieves wiped the drive clean without even looking at what it contained; since then, she has become somewhat of an expert in data encryption.

How to Record Your Orgasm for Your Lover

 HOTTEST!

One way to way to stoke the fire—and be sexy as hell—is to let your lover hear your orgasm when he or she can't be with you. Whether it's a normal workday or a weeklong business trip, sending them an orgasm by MP3 is a creative way to show how you feel.

Sharing an audio orgasm is not only erotic, it shows the recipient just how deeply you trust the file won't show up on a blog or make the rounds of email—unless you don't mind if it does.

★ Gather whatever you need for your solo play: lube, sex toys, scented candles, special blanket, erotic novel, or magazine.

★ If you have a laptop, you can record in your bed or wherever else you are comfortable. If you have a desktop in the kitchen, make a nest of pillows and blankets on the floor and choose a time when you are sure that you will be left alone long enough to complete the mission.

★ Plug in your computer microphone. Headsets are nice because they put the mic right near your lips but leave your hands free. If that makes you shy, or if you have music going and you want your moans and breath to be less prominent in the result, you can set the mic by your side.

★ Open your recording software. I use Audacity, a free audio editing application available at audacity.sourceforge.net. You can also record using your iPod with a mic attachment, a cell phone or PDA with a "voice memo" feature, or in a pinch, leave yourself a voicemail. (Sign up for a GotVoice account at www.gotvoice.com to download your voicemails from your phone to your computer for sharing.)

★ Test your microphone: Click Record and try some heavy breathing, turn the vibrator on for a few seconds, adjust the volume on the music. Capture about 20 seconds, then click Stop. Click Play to hear what you've got. If the mic didn't pick up your breathing, move it closer to your head. Repeat the test a few times until you get the levels you want.

★ Settle in and click Record.

★ Do your solo. It doesn't matter how long it takes, so forget about the recording and just have a good time. Your lover would much rather hear your genuine experience than a fake performance.

★ When you're finished, wipe your hands off and click Stop.

★ Save the file in a safe place where you won't accidentally launch it during a work presentation.

★ When you play it back, you might feel self-conscious or silly or embarrassed, but don't. Our orgasm sounds, just like our orgasm faces, are precious to our lovers, even if we squirm when we hear them ourselves.

★ You want a clip of 2–3 minutes, so find the part where things really heat up. Generally this will be toward the end, when your breathing speeds up and your moans and cries are more frequent.

★ Highlight this section with the mouse.

★ From the File menu, click Export Selection to MP3. (This works in Audacity. If you use another audio program, find its instructions for editing your file and saving it as an MP3.) MP3 is a common format that everyone can play, so it's a good choice for sharing.

★ At the prompt, enter a name for the MP3 file.

★ Send the MP3 file to your lover with a note explaining what it is. I wouldn't risk keeping the contents a surprise unless you don't mind his friends or coworkers overhearing it when he launches the file, thinking it's a song.

I don't recommend putting the file on your lover's iPod or computer without their knowledge. You never know when they will have their songs on Shuffle with other people around.

How to Have Even More Fun with Your Audio Vibrator

HOTTEST!

Remember the joy of the mix tape, crafted especially for you by that special someone? Sound-sensitive vibrators offer a variation for adults only, as the devices pulse, rev, and throb to the beat of audio sources ranging from a music playlist to your lover's voice.

If you've read "How to Turn Your MP3 Player into a Personal Pleasure Device" on page 19, you're already on the right track. These tips will get you in the groove for using these special gadgets together with your partner.

★ Make a special playlist for you or your lover's portable music player, choosing songs that have the right combination of emotional expression and stimulating vibration.

★ Meet up in a virtual club in Second Life, Red Light Center, or another 3D world, and plug your vibrators into your computer headphone jacks. (Great for groups!)

★ Talk to your lover over Skype, Yahoo, or other audio chat program, and let your voices drive the vibrations.

★ Pop some audio erotica into the CD player, plug in the vibrator, and enjoy an extra touch to the stories.

★ Watch a naughty movie with the vibe plugged in and discover a whole new purpose for the ridiculous "bonk-chica-bow" music.

★ For a special occasion, create a multimedia experience out of video, pictures, and song. Package it with an audio toy, scented candle, flavored lube, and lingerie, and you'll arouse all the senses.

★ For a private thrill in public, tuck a bullet vibe into your underpants and keep your music source in your pocket. Let everyone wonder why you can't keep the smile off your face. And try not to squirm.

How to Have Satisfying Erotic Instant Message Sessions

HOTTEST!

Instant message comes naturally to me and has been the platform of many a delicious conversation, from explicit flirting to three-hour cybersex sessions. But it doesn't just happen on its own. It takes more than fast fingers to transform IM from a text window on the screen to an escape into delicious sexual fantasy.

★ Adjust the atmosphere in the room. Dim the lights, make the chair comfortable, light candles. (Extra points for buying candles in the same scent as your lover's and burning them together.)

★ If you know each other well enough to mail things (or trade them when you see each other), exchange clothing that holds your scents, and wear it or drape it close by when you IM.

★ Open the IM window to a comfortable size and adjust the font type, size, and color to something easy on your eyes.

★ Clear the clutter off your desk so it doesn't distract your imagination. At least hide the bills and the inbox. If things get slow, you don't want to be tempted to take care of business on the side.

★ Close and lock your door if you live with other people. Better yet, give them movie passes and lock the front door behind them.

★ Keep a clean towel handy.

★ If you like sex toys, keep them handy too.

★ Let your imagination run wild. Think of all the words, all the ways you can go, the freedom you have, because it's IM and you have to be as vivid as possible in just . . . words.

★ Collect words as you go through life, seeking new ways to put an erotic spin on everyday language. Think dirty, uncommon, slang, literary, high-falutin', and multilingual—for starters.

How to Remain Sexually Active Through Injury, Disability, or Pain

HOTTEST!

Chronic pain depresses the libido and creates obstacles to desire and pleasure. Both pain and medication make a person exhausted; chronic pain often causes depression, frustration, and anger, which can add strain to the relationship on a number of levels, including sex. And while sex helps with relaxation and even eases pain—I have a friend who uses it for relief from migraine headaches—it's hard to drum up desire when you're already stressed and tired.

And yet, couples do find ways to work with the limitations of a lover's injury, illness, or disability.

Every person experiences pain differently, just like every person's sexuality is unique. It's impossible to recommend any single solution for individuals or couples trying to keep sexual intimacy in their lives, but these tips can help you get started.

★ Even if a partner wants to engage physically, an extremely sensitive neurological system can inhibit the pleasure response. A touch that feels ticklish or mildly tender on most people might be excruciating to a person with, say, fibromyalgia. In this situation, tantra can be key. This is more than just touching each other's foreheads and thinking pure, loving thoughts. It is an intense form of communication in which you stare deep into each other's eyes and learn what it means when a nerve jumps or a muscle twitches or a breath catches in your throat.

★ Replace the goal of orgasm with the goal of pleasuring the partner with the pain condition. The more a person can feel pleasure instead of pain, the more likely the libido will rise to the occasion.

★ Be aware that you might be causing pain when you intend to create pleasure. Tune into your lover's body and breath, and focus on being empathic.

★ Furniture and devices designed to facilitate sex can help. Look into Liberator shapes, the Monkey Rocker, the Body Bouncer, the Bonkum, or even the Sybian for interesting ways to support bodies and provide stimulation (perhaps for the partner who isn't in pain). For people with increased sensitivity, a very gentle massager like the Happy Kitty, which uses a push–pull suction mechanism rather than rapid side-to-side vibration, can provide stimulation without being overwhelming. The one-time-use vibrating rings available in the condom section of the local drugstore (well, in most states) can also provide a little oomph.

★ Medical-grade vacuum pumps and vasoconstrictor rings that help men get and sustain erections are available by prescription. Sex and disability expert Cory Silverberg says the less expensive models available at quality adult retailers are less ergonomic but work just as well.

★ Experiment, let go of shyness, and get creative with how you use things. A vibrating sleeve made for a penis can feel good on a forearm, too. A person who can't stand the feel of a feather on her skin might enjoy something percussive, like a paddle.

★ Don't stop talking about sex. The partner in pain might lose interest in sex and get angry and frustrated at the other's "demands" for intimacy. Or the hurt partner might feel alienated, unattractive, or useless. If a person feels they can no longer have positive sensual or physical experience in their lives, they tend to withdraw, and then the other person stops trying to initiate sex. No one wants to feel like they are pressuring their lover for intimacy, and neither partner enjoys a pattern of rejection. But there are ways to be compassionate through it all. "I wish I did want to have sex, but I don't" is honest and gentle and opens the door to talking about ways you can be intimate without having sex.

★ Expand your definition of sex. Sex can be a lot of different things, from looking at erotic content together while stroking each other's skin to whispering fantasies in each other's ears to playing an online erotic game. One person can tell a story while the other masturbates. Massage oils, lubes, erotic audio books, dildos on bouncing balls, sleeves, raunchy email and IM conversations, cock rings, and—I've recently discovered—French lessons on the MP3 player are all capable of adding both excitement and adaptability to sexual activity.

★ Honor that sexuality is important in the relationship.

★ For unexplained pain, talk to health practitioners about diet and lifestyle changes. Avoiding gluten (wheat) and soy has alleviated or even eliminated fibromyalgia symptoms in some folks. Natural health advocates usually recommend avoiding artificial sweeteners and all stimulants, including caffeine, guarana, and echinacea. If massage or acupuncture help, make sure to find a body worker who understands the person's goals with the treatment.

★ Progressive doctors will sometimes recommend a brief vacation from medication, just a few days, to let the libido bounce back enough for sex.

★ Remember that the brain is the most important sex organ. If you can have a meeting of the minds, you can share erotic experiences.

How to Give Good Word

HOTTER!

Even in 3D environments and webcam chat rooms, the heart of cybersex is storytelling, and the way most people do that is still through text. That's one of the reasons cybersex is so popular among women—we love a good story, and those of us who spend a lot of time online often do so because we respond so well to words. A wordsmith who can arouse us is a wordsmith we want to get to know better, someone we want to match fire for fire.

These tips aren't going to transform you into a world-class erotica writer overnight, but that's only because great prose, like great sex, can't be rushed. Refer to "How to Publish Your Sexy Story" on page 98 for more information on what you can do with words once you start wielding them.

★ Don't use over-the-top romance novel language like "manroot" or "member" unless you really mean it and are using those words for effect.

★ Give and take the lead, following the other person's language at times and then guiding them toward yours at other times.

YOUR PERSONAL WORD LIST

This is just a short list of some words to keep handy for cybersex. Many of these are more porno than erotic, and it is by no means an exhaustive list. Don't be too quick to cross off the words you hate—you never know how it's going to feel when you use it for the first time in contact. But do grab a pen and add all the words you can think of that suit your erotic imagination.

There. See how easy that was, given a place to start?

NOUNS

Ass	Juice
Asshole	Length
Back door	Lips
Balls	Member
Blow job	Mons
Box	Organ
Butt	Penis
Button	Perineum
Clit	Pussy
Cock	Sac
Come	Shaft
Cream	Slit
Cunt	Snatch
Curves	Teeth
Dick	Testicles
Fingers/	Thigh
fingertips	Tongue
Hair	Trail of hair
Head	Twat
Hole	Vagina
Honey	Vulva

VERBS

Bind	Go down	Rock
Bite	Handcuff	Rub
Blow	Hump	Shout
Breathe	Jut	Slap
Bury	Kiss	Spank
Come	Lave	Speak
Control	Lick	Suck
Cream	Moan	Swell
Cry out	Nibble	Talk
Drip	Pant	Taste
Eat	Pinch	Tease
Enclose	Plunge	Tempt
Engulf	Possess	Throb
Enter	Pound	Thrust
Entwine	Pulse/	Tie
Finger	pulsate	Touch
Flick	Pump	Whimper
Fuck	Put	Whip
Give head	Ride	

ADJECTIVES/ADVERBS

Bad	Long
Deep	Look/watch
Dripping	Red/pink/
Firm/firmly	other colors
Good	Sexy
Hard	Soft/softly
Horny	Stiff
Hot	Strong
Juicing	Swollen
Jutting	Tireless
Lightly	Wet

★ Keep a list of alternative words handy. Good writers know the value of the thesaurus. It's like a vibrating ring for your lexicon.

★ Jot down juicy phrases and acts during the day as you think of them, so if you're on the spot at midnight with that hot Australian, you have something to whip out. So to speak.

★ Offer variety. Although the sexual connection is real, the environment is fantasy in the sense that it is not bound by the usual rules of gravity, balance, or proportion. Let that free your mind (and the rest will follow).

★ Dare to step outside your comfort zone and explore sexual activities you haven't done, and think you wouldn't do if you were offline.

★ Joke, banter, and play. "Adult" communities aren't just for sex, and in fact, most of the conversation that takes place is not direct cybersex. But these are spaces where we can let our minds roam free, without worry of offending the people around us. Social expectations of ladylike behavior need not constrain our senses of humor.

★ Think about the kinds of conversation you like to have before, during, and after sex. Cyberspace gives you the opportunity to learn to initiate and have that intercourse, and that's a skill that doesn't have to stay relegated to online lovin'.

How to Find Out
Whether You Are Kinky

HOTTEST!

One thing we've learned from each other in the information age is that kinky is as kinky does. What we used to think was only us—in delight or in shame—we now find is not unique at all.

Think of how society is going to change in the next ten years as we realize we are not alone in our desires. Of course, this new openness can be frustrating if you're someone who needs to feel avant-garde to get excited.

As "kinky" comes to mean any form of sex beyond the most vanilla*, it's not so much a matter of finding out *whether* you are kinky as finding out *how* kinky you are. Kinky does not mean you have a fetish or an obsession, only that a particular flavor of sex—involving props, theater, groups of people, public places, etc.—can pretty much be relied upon to get you excited.

You can expand your knowledge of your own kinks online in a few ways.

★ When stumbling across a kink in porn, you realize you're turned on. Now, go find more porn featuring that quirk and discover whether it affects you consistently.

★ Research a particular kink from your own fantasies—from something you've experienced once or twice and liked, or from books or movies that introduced you to that whole new world.

★ Get involved in a community based around a kink. This could be as simple as a message board or chat room, or as involved as a Second Life group in which members meet twice a month in-world and attend an annual real-life meet-up.

★ Hire an escort in a virtual world to help you explore.

★ Visit a webcam room that caters to a particular kink or fetish, like latex, balloons, leather, or BDSM.

★ Read or listen to erotica that you wouldn't normally choose and see if it arouses you.

★ Search your city—or a destination city, if you're traveling—for kink-related parties and events open to newbies. Many sex groups have regular dinners where people can come and talk to the members and learn more about the scene. A good place to start is http://eros-zine.com.

★ Many adult retailers offer classes in the basics and post their workshop calendars online. Because some kink can hurt you if you do it wrong—for example, there are safe and unsafe ways to bind somebody—it's always better to get information from an expert first.

---

* Vanilla is as vague of a term as kinky, and can mean anything from "heterosexual missionary position" to "anything just involving bodies; no toys or porn or costumes." The only objection kinky people have to vanilla sex is when people who believe vanilla sex should be the only permitted sexual activity try to set rules and even laws for everyone else.

How to Find Out
Whether Your Lover Is Kinky

HOTTEST!

Anything you want to know about your lover you should be able to ask. But what if the answer is "I don't know?!" or even *"Eeek! No! Never! Of course not! How could you even think—how could you* ask *me that? Ugh!"*

If you learned through the Internet that you are kinky—a word which today means "interested in more than vanilla sex, although we're not sure now where to draw the line between vanilla and other flavors" (is anal considered vanilla by now?)—you are probably now wondering whether your partner will join you in your new explorations.

One way to find out, obviously, is to talk about your own discoveries, and what it means to you not just as part of your sexuality but as part of your life as a whole. Another is to bring them along with you as you explore.

★ Send your partner a link to content that turned you on and ask for an opinion.

★ Start including tastes of your discoveries in email, text messages, and IM, and wait for a response. If it's positive, turn up the heat.

★ Introduce your lover to Stockroom.com and ExtremeRestraints.com, and then wonder aloud whether it might be fun to find a third party to come over and teach the two of you about domination and submission.

★ If you find something you really want, and your partner objects and won't try, what then? Can you satisfy it online? How important is it? Can you meet each other halfway?

★ Invite your partner to a kink workshop—maybe even build a weekend trip around it, and do the class in another city.

How to Control a
Sex Toy over the Internet

HOTTEST!

While mainly used by long-distance lovers and frequent travelers, Internet-enabled sex toys can also be naughty fun when one of you is at the office and the other is in the boudoir. Known by the rather unromantic name of "teledildonics," this field has been struggling to reach its market for years. Yet even as legal issues surrounding trademarks and patents have held back the commercialization of adult Internet appliances, developers are continuing to push the technology forward.

Lillian Yiyuan, a writer and a Second Life club owner, is working on Bluetooth-enabled toys that interface with Second Life. Robotics engineer Kyle Machulis oversees the Opendildonics project, which encourages developers to create and share open-source code that anyone can use to build their own systems.

At press time, consumers had a few off-the-shelf products to try.

HIGHJOY.COM

The HighJoy system uses Doc Johnson toys—a rabbit pearl vibrator for women and a sleeve with a vibrating bullet for men. You buy the toy and subscribe to the service in order to have access to the connection software. (The toys require a serial port; if your computer doesn't have one, don't forget to buy the serial-to-USB adapter when you place your order.) Each partner gets a control panel that adjusts the pattern, intensity, and speed of the other's toy. The chat program supports audio and video, as well as text.

SINULATOR

The Sinulator (http://sinulate.com) has an advantage over HighJoy in that it is wireless. You plug the transmitter into a USB port and then take the toy wherever you like (within range). The controller on your toy can be switched over to control your partner's toy. If your bed is out of range of your webcam but you want to add video to the experience, you can always invest in a set of Ojo video phones (www.ojophone.com).

VIRTUAL SEX MACHINE

At press time, this intriguing machine was available only for men; I list it here because it might be a fun way to surprise your guy on his birthday and because the developers have talked about developing a similar device for women. While at first the thing looks scary, I can see why it has been a successful product—the first time I slipped my fingers inside the demo model, I wished they made something like this for massaging feet and hands. It truly feels wonderful, and the suction and stimulation mechanisms are impressive. To use it, a man plugs the toy into his computer and plays one of the specially encoded DVDs. The DVD sends signals to the device, controlling its motions based on what's going on in the video. Most of the videos are shot in "first person," so the man can pretend the woman on the screen is doing wonderful things to him, and that he is doing wonderful things to her. See http://vrinnovations.com.

Now see the lesson, "How to Get the Most out of Teledildonics" on page 236, for some tips on getting off to a smooth start.

How to Pick the Best Type of Lover

 HOT!

This one's easy. Find a geek.

1. GEEKS BUILD IT SO YOU WILL COME.

Second Life's SexGen animation system, Red Light Center's beautiful sex animations, and open-source teledildonics did not simply coalesce out of the mists during a marketing department meeting.

These types of projects require strong technical know-how along with an open-minded approach to sexual variation. After all, you can't build sex-tech that serves only your own preferences if you expect others to use it. Especially if you want them to buy it.

That geeks have the passion to commit their technical skills to expanding sexual options for everyone is evidence enough of their enthusiasm and dedication as lovers.

2. GEEKS BIND TO TECH IN PERSONAL WAYS.

All engineers may be geeks, but not all geeks are engineers. Doesn't matter. You don't need to know how to build a platform in order to do a half-gainer in full pike with a twist into the river of love.

A geek is more likely to figure out how to customize toys and to design arousing environments for your avatars to play in than a nongeek. And that experience translates into a greater sensitivity to atmosphere and mood during sex—beyond just lighting a candle.

Don't be surprised if your geek lover puts more thought into arranging the boudoir than you do, or if common household items ("pervertibles") soon take on a new dimension. More than one geek has told me that Home Depot is their favorite adult store.

3. GEEKS SLIP EASILY INTO CONSENSUAL ROLE PLAYING.

Geek lovers combine a well-developed and oft-exercised erotic imagination with their physical technique. It isn't a big leap from "I'm a level-13 thief, evil-aligned" to "I'm the prison warden, and you're the new detainee." Scientists and therapists alike claim that the brain is the most critical sexual organ; a geek's familiarity with fantasy arouses your mind even as the handcuffs—or the bag of loot—bring your body to attention.

4. GEEKS INTERACT.

Where a technophobe is able to talk to you in person, a geek is also happy to be with you by texting your phone, flirting with you in a chat room, Skyping you, Twittering just in case you're on your vibrating couch, sending funny cell phone snapshots to your email, playing online games, commenting on your blog, digging up articles that interest you, seducing you by instant message . . . .

5. GEEKS GET THINGS DONE.

Geeks know all the shortcuts. Geek lovers can research your interests, send you surprise gifts, plan your perfect vacation, get the bills and grocery shopping out of the way, write to their mothers, and tease you mercilessly, all while pretending to work. And when you ask them to set up your home's Wi-Fi or install a home theater, it's done quickly, expertly, and without complaint.

In other words, geeks know how to get everything else out of the way so there's more time for lovemaking.

6. GEEKS ARE HOT . . .

. . . and wear the coolest glasses.

7. GEEKS DON'T SHOCK EASILY.

Geeks have seen all the porn you can imagine and then some, priming them to be open to your sexual idiosyncracies. Geeks are not only less likely to be shocked by your exotic requests—they might not even realize that other people think your turn-ons are exotic. In fact, your geek lover might be relieved that your wildest fantasy involves only two other people, five utensils, and a trapeze.

8. GEEKS KNOW KINKY PEOPLE.

Geeks haven't just seen a variety of positions, kinks, and fetishes in blue movies. Geeks know (or are) people who enjoy those things, so they don't dismiss entire categories of sexual interests as the sole province of a bunch of weirdos in San Francisco.

It's hard to sustain prejudice and bias against an abstract group when you develop relationships with individuals and discover they're just like you. It doesn't matter if they dress up like ponies, or refuse to conform to a societal idea of gender norms, or eat pancakes for dinner. Geek lovers know better than to try to impose their sexual preferences or standards on others—including your friends—and are more likely to love and let love.

9. GEEKS UNDERSTAND MULTIDIMENSIONAL RELATIONSHIPS.

Geeks connect with their online buddies in several guises, often getting to know the person behind the avatar as friendships deepen and move from adult communities to personal IM.

A geek can flow seamlessly between conversation about a friend's partner and kids in one window and an elaborate group sex scene in another, without feeling any discontinuity between the personas—even if the friend is a forty-three-year-old father of two in IM but a twenty-two-year-old dominatrix in the group.

With all that going on, a geek has no problem accepting that sometimes you want mocha ripple cherry fudge chunk swirl with almonds and a waffle, and sometimes you want vanilla lite.

10. GEEKS AREN'T EASILY THREATENED BY NEW TECH OR "THE FUTURE OF SEX."

A geek doesn't mind if you bring home the iiErotoTrix 5000 v3—as long as you share it.

Geeks have read the science fiction. Geeks know the dire predictions of a world in which the sticky press of flesh is replaced by neural nets and sex robots that also do housework (or house robots that also do sex work).

Geeks have imagined more sexual dystopias than the average person and are the first to see the technological developments that could lead us down dark paths. And geeks know better than anyone that something always goes wrong when you lean on machines for all of your social fulfillment.

Literacy and the printing press did not replace sex; neither did photography, automobiles, video, online porn, or 3D escort services. Geek lovers spend enough time with technology to appreciate the unique wondrousness of human touch.

How to Laugh Your Way Through Technical Difficulties and into Great Webcam Sex

HOTTEST!

"Is yours on?"

"There it is."

"Oh! It's working!"

"Shoot. Frozen again."

"Let's try a different cam program."

"Can you see me now?"

"Crap. Wait. Is that . . . did I get it?"

"Ah ha! There you are!"

That might not sound like foreplay to you, but even in these modern times, it's an all too common way to begin a webcam session. By the time you fix the connection, the camera, the lighting, the angle, and the audio, any romantic mood is long past. And when it's finally all working, you sit there, gazing dazedly at one another, wondering what to say and how to recapture the moment.

The best thing you can do is laugh. Release those tech-induced tensions and take delight in your ability to work through a frustrating experience

BY GOLLY, IT JUST MIGHT WORK

Here's the webcam setup that I have had the best luck with:

★ Broadband Internet connection

★ Ethernet cable (rather than wireless)

★ Skype video chat software (if the connection is unstable, stop the call and restart until you get a solid picture)

★ A better-than-bargain webcam ($50 and up)

★ A good headset with microphone (which will be better than the webcam's built-in mic)

together. Then write down exactly what you did—any programs, settings, and workarounds you added that fixed the problems. You never know, it might actually help get things together faster in your next session.

It's especially important to accept setbacks like this with equanimity, especially if you only have so much time to be together before your privacy will be interrupted. Otherwise, your memory of the session will be tarnished with negative emotion rather than the joy that you managed to carve out some time.

If you have the whole night ahead, relax, laugh, and when the mood starts to lift, take it where you originally intended. A come-hither facial expression and the solemn removal of an article of clothing is an effective way to regain focus.

How to Create a
Mobile Sex Shuttle

HOTTER!

I'm now in my mid-thirties. But I am apparently making up for a teenagehood that barely involved any making out or sex in cars. And maybe it's because of my age that I've taken care to outfit my truck bed for maximum pleasure, creating a true love nest on wheels with all the modern conveniences.

Furniture specifically designed for lovemaking is your best bet—much more comfortable and conducive to good sex than an old sleeping bag or blanket. It also transforms the space into a private alcove for snuggling, reading, and talking.

★ Buy a truck with at least a six-foot bed.

★ Add a camper shell that has darkly tinted windows.

★ Lay the foundation: Purchase a lovemaking pad from Liberator, made from a special foam so it gives you cushioned support where you want it and provides a moisture-proof surface for easy clean-up.

CAUTION

Car sex is an American tradition dating back at least a hundred years, but be careful. In some states, getting caught canoodling in the car can lead to prosecution and a listing in the sex offender database, depending on whether a citizen files a complaint—or makes a citizen's arrest—and what kind of mood the police officer is in. In a remote location, you might get away with a knock on the window and a "move along, kids." But in a public venue like a city park, in broad daylight, while kids on field trips come out to feed the ducks? You might want to keep your clothes on and stick to good old-fashioned necking.

★ Add luxury: Invest in a Liberator wedge for resting your heads on as you lie side by side, and for use under your (or your lover's) hips to aid in positioning. A throw pillow or two can make a nice nesting spot too. Just make sure not to add so many that you can't fit your lover in there with you.

★ Add warmth: Buy sturdy bedding. Here's where the blankets and sleeping bags come in, or if you want to splurge, the sheets designed for lovemaking. These are good if your truck bed isn't watertight, like mine—the moisture-resistant fabrics repel any rain that trickles in through the tailgate.

★ Add pleasure: A duffel bag looks unassuming to a casual glance through the window, but it can hold a collection of toys, erotic novels, nipple jewelry, floggers, and other interesting paraphernalia just as easily as gym clothes.

You can keep lube and towels in here too, but be careful about keeping condoms in the truck, as excessive heat can weaken the material and make them more prone to breakage.

✔ Scout out locations: If you have an Inspiration Point or Makeout Rock handy, you're ahead of the game. You want to find places where you can be discreet yet safe—no abandoned warehouses in the rough part of town, for example. Parks are traditional and safe for necking; for more than heavy petting, you'll want to be somewhere less likely to attract families and police officers. Also, park in the shade. Bright sunlight will make you wonder if the window tinting helps at all.

✔ Stay within your comfort zone. If the thought of being seen by the security guard at the parking garage freezes you up and you can't find anywhere private enough to ease your heart, try your own driveway.

How to Have Aural Sex

HOTTER!

Aural sex is a wonderful way to get close to someone.
In fact, it's so intimate, some women are more shy about phone sex than physical sex!

Of course, aural sex is no longer tied to the phone. We have all kinds of opportunities to give voice to our sexual fantasies, with our one special someone or with a group. Mobile phones free us from having to be anywhere in particular in order to have a conversation; Skype frees us to talk with anyone in the world—for free if they have Internet and for very cheap if you have to call their phone.

> *Resist the temptation to shout, even into a cell phone. A gentle, quiet, focused voice helps the other person's brain filter out distractions and focus on you.*
>
> —Midori, sex educator and author

★ Figure out how long your lover's voicemail lets you talk, and then call it and tell him a story. A sexy story. A story so hot that when the beep sounds and cuts you off, your lover is panting for more. You can also read your lover stories or serialize an erotic novel for them over time, leaving one or more days between installments so they never know when they're going to get the next bit.

★ Record a love note, save it to MP3 and email it. See "How to Record Your Orgasm for Your Lover" on page 202 for technical tips.

★ Buy a headphone splitter so you can listen to the same audio device together. One trick is to listen to erotic stories while stroking and petting—and then pull his headphones out at a critical moment. Before he has a chance to feel bereft, pick up where the story left off. You know what I mean.

★ Audio is a great venue for role playing. Midori, a sex educator based in San Francisco who teaches aural sex workshops all around the world, says that in role playing, couples often overcome self-consciousness. They return to that sense of play and mutual permission for the suspension of disbelief that they had as children. And then they combine that with the "fundamental libidinous self."

★ Slow down, keep your voice sweet and sexy and quiet. Aural sex is a chance to step out of the fast pace of modern life, and you should give yourself enough time to get comfortable with the mode. Remember that your partner can't see you, so you need to put into words those things you otherwise let your body say for you.

★ Practice using silence. Listen to each other breathe. You can hear someone smile through the phone, even if they're not talking.

★ Play with rich, sensory descriptions, and don't be afraid to take chances.

★ Slow it down; don't be afraid of moments of silence. Instead of being loud, use a quiet, focused voice.

★ The human brain focuses in on soft sounds the way a dog's ears swivel to catch the slightest nuance of a noise, but it's often hard to distinguish words over the phone if you talk softly. If you whisper, speak more slowly so your lover can understand you without asking you to repeat anything.

★ Some people have resisted the use of voice technology in virtual worlds, arguing that allowing people to use audio chat destroys the fantasy with too much reality. And yet, our voices provide such a powerful way for humans to connect that lovers who spend time together in virtual worlds will often connect by voice through another medium, such as cell phones or instant message, while they are in-world. To put a twist on mom's advice about not talking smack about others: If you have something sexy to say, say it.

How to Get the Most out of Teledildonics

HOTTEST!

Some people like the thrill of giving up control of their vibrator to their partner or online lovers. Others like the extra layer of communication these intimate interfaces require, as you both have to talk to each other about what you want, what feels good, and what you could do without.

And still others like the chance to be an exhibitionist, voyeur, or both—all without leaving the house (and often without exposing your face).

Whatever your reasons for buying a teledildonics system, these tips will help you get the most out of your investment.

★ If you feel silly, laugh; if you feel self-conscious, enjoy it. When was the last time you got all shy and squirmy with your partner?

★ If you expect technical difficulties, they won't blast your mood to shards when they arise. (You're more likely to have trouble with your webcam connections than with your teledildonics system.)

★ Have a contingency plan for network problems. All of the Internet-enabled toys also work fine as stand-alone vibrators, so if you have to control it yourself while you talk on the phone, you can always try the Internet again another night.

★ Keep spare batteries on hand. After you get everything plugged in, the Internet connection working, the webcams steady, the voice connection strong, the cords out of the way or the wireless receiver within range . . . the last thing you need is for the batteries to die.

★ Don't expect the experience (or the technology) to be more than it is. Accept that it's a fun way to play, and don't be disappointed when it's not the same as in-person sex. That's okay—it's not meant to be a replacement.

How to Take Your Online Discoveries Offline

HOTTEST!

You might want to put on your seatbelt—or other handy safety gear—as this is a big one.

Playing online can teach you all kinds of wonderful, delicious things about yourself and your sexuality. And if you're like most people, you will eventually begin to hunger for more. What seemed daring in the privacy of your cool dark room now seems old hat, as quotidian as a soy latte and a Sudoku puzzle.

We take our online discoveries into the offline world in several ways. Many times, we can't help the transfer from happening—or might not even notice when it does. The change might be in the form of a new sexual confidence, a better sense of what we want, or a willingness to engage in difficult conversations in the pursuit of deeper intimacy or greater harmony within a relationship.

Everything we learn about our fantasies and desires infuses all of our romantic and sexual relationships. Yet sometimes it's challenging to consciously make that transition once the buffer of the Internet is taken away and we're looking our partners in the eye (or casting our eyes downward at their feet) and mumbling that we want them to spank us, tie us up, or take us in the ass.

Or all three, all at once. And even in today's modern world, many people will probably, and perhaps justifiably, get nervous if you tell them, "Oh, don't worry, I practiced this online." Especially if you have a strap-on harness and a nine-inch dildo in your hands.

Here are some guidelines for merging the confidence and open boundaries of online play into your offline play without overwhelming other people with your forthrightness.

★ If you've had good relationships with people online, you've probably learned to communicate clearly and continuously. When it comes time to have difficult conversations offline, you can draw on that experience and think of how you would say it in chat or IM. And then just say it. If you've been playing in adult spaces online, tone it down offline. I went through a few months where the most inappropriate innuendos slipped from my lips, and where I had an almost constant leer in mixed company. Once you get used to total verbal freedom, it's frustrating to rein it in. You want to be as witty as you are in your online community, and to command the same level of attention—but it just makes you seem odd, coming on three times stronger than you should around new people. If you can catch half the "mature" content before it flies out of your mouth, you will still have a reputation as a sexually open, confident being. And you'll help avoid the wrong kind of attention.

★ Have patience with those around you. Your girlfriends may not recognize the unleashed you. New and potential lovers might be bowled over by your enthusiasm. Your ability to accept sexual variations, now that you've seen everything and done most of it online, is wonderful and inclusive, and people will be less afraid to share that part of themselves with you. At the same time, taking a paramour home for the first time and surprising them with your brand-new homemade dungeon only works if you've already talked about BDSM ahead of time. Otherwise, start 'em on more familiar ground and let them get used to you.

★ Accept that time moves slower in meatspace, and enjoy the wait. In a chat room, women who like to get sexy (verbally or on camera) are often mobbed. In a nightclub, it's not so obvious. At the coffee-and-cookies hour after a religious service? A raised eyebrow is about the best you can expect. And he's probably married anyway. If you remember that time, and relationships, move much faster online, you'll be better prepared to enjoy the slower pace of deliberate, physical seduction offline.

★ Respect your partner's worries. If your partner knows you've been playing around online, it's possible that he or she will feel some concern. After all, many, many people who don't intend to do more than play wind up falling head over heels for the idealized person they meet, with disastrous effects on the existing relationship. But if your relationship is strong and communicative, and especially if you are exploring the new world together, you can greatly enrich your sex life by bringing your newfound understandings—and interests—into real-time.

★ Your lover is probably going to be delighted that you've become more adventurous in bed. Cybersex tends to help us shed fears that used to hold us back, and since we get used to exercising our erotic brains, we don't let our bodies get in our way as much. If you start to worry that you look silly or unattractive, pretend you're cybering, and just let it go.

★ Chat rooms and virtual worlds might have you hooked on the group thing. Did you know that this is pretty common stuff offline too? You'll find swinger clubs in lots of places you didn't think they'd exist, and big cities have sex parties and erotic events galore. Eros Zine (http://eros-zine.com) has club event listings; http://sexuality.org has an extensive guide to group and swinging sex.

★ Many people discover polyamory for the first time through their online play. For some, it is possible to be truly in love with more than one person at a time. Franklin Veaux maintains an excellent resource at http://xeromag.com where you can learn about the many variations of polyamory, the challenges of bringing polyamory into a formerly monogamous relationship, and the emotional risks and rewards of stepping outside societal assumptions about the "right way" to partner.

★ Online explorations can open our minds and hearts to sexuality in surprising ways. In some cases, a partner might resist or even feel threatened by the changes he or she senses in you. If you have a good relationship with your partner and want to keep it that way, find ways to help him or her get comfortable with the sexy new you.

★ If what you've discovered is that you need to leave the relationship and move on, and you know that for sure, do so with faith in yourself—and with integrity. You aren't the first woman for whom Internet relating has been the catalyst to a new and better life. It almost always involves a lot of pain and heartbreak, but a long, slow death of a relationship that cannot be salvaged involves more.

How to Take Your First Step into BDSM

HOTTEST!

I don't know if it's just me, but BDSM seems to be everywhere these days. (Yay!) BDSM stands for Bondage and Discipline (BD), Dominance and Submission (DS), Sadism and Masochism (SM), and it sums up a wide spectrum of activity, from gentle bondage through eroticized (and consensual) torture.

It makes sense that BDSM is so popular online. For one thing, many people start with fantasy long before they venture into acting it out, and the interactive environment lets you engage with another person and see how you like it without literally being flogged or punished.

Another thing is that BDSM is very theatrical, very visual. It gives erotic designers an opportunity to challenge their skills, building sets and implements and costumes and environments in 3D worlds for themselves and for others.

Much of the erotica available online brushes up against or outright embraces BDSM. Nothing like pain and pleasure combined to add drama to a romantic, sexual, or erotic story.

LEARNING THE ROPES

One friend of mine got his first-aid certification as part of his journey into more extreme BDSM practices. Another took two workshops in rope bondage before trying it on his partner in a private setting. Please invest the time and research into learning to play safely. Not every escort or partner in an online community knows what they're doing. But when you take it into physical space you can actually place yourself in physical danger if you don't know what you're doing. There are places on the body it is dangerous to flog, there are dangerous ways to bind people, and there are chances for accidents, like starting fires or causing internal injury. Playing it safe (heh) is *fun,* will enhance your experience, and could save your life.

All in all, online BDSM communities welcome the chance to introduce newbies into safe, sane play. Several escorts in virtual worlds cater specifically to the curious and the inexperienced.

To do BDSM right, you need to follow some basic safety guidelines; these not only pertain to your physical health, but to your emotional, spiritual, and mental well-being as well.

Alt.com, an online dating/social networking site for kinky people, has a good collection of articles in its Magazine section that will introduce you to the principles behind safe play. Sexuality.org and http://xeromag.com also offer extensive BDSM information, while http://bondage.com has a "BDSM U" for members and a Q&A column available to nonmembers.

How to Manage a Harem Online

HOTTEST!

The Internet has given millions of people a taste of what it's like to have more than one lover at a time. For some, this means being deeply in love with more than one partner. For others, it means having a primary partner and then other lovers on a more casual basis. And for others, it means having multiple partners of varying levels of affection and commitment. But even in fantasy, having many lovers can create logistical problems. Love might be infinite, but time is not.

And then there is the etiquette. Do you introduce them to each other or not? Do you know about their other lovers or not? Do you open several IM windows simultaneously for your birthday, or do you pull them all into a group chat for extra special fun? The answer to all of these questions is "maybe." You have to figure out what works for you.

Most people don't go online for exclusivity. Part of the reason we're there is to explore, which generally means logging on when we can and talking to lots of people. Every relationship is different, so I can't tell you exactly how to balance your lovers and give each relationship what it needs. But you can apply these general principles to every situation.

★ Respect your partners.

★ Don't demand more time than they can give you, and don't turn yourself inside out trying to be online for someone every moment of every day. If you're exhausted, you won't be an able or a willing partner.

★ Competitiveness just causes headaches. You might treat the relationship like a time-share (everyone has certain time set aside for online dates) or a co-op (everyone is welcome and knows each other), but if you treat it like a winner-takes-all endurance race, you're going to lose.

★ Learn from real-life polyamorous groups. See http://sexuality.org and http://xeromag.com for a practical look at the different ways poly people work.

★ Some people use different names, or "alts," when spending time with different lovers. It's a way to keep things organized, as well as to distinguish between ongoing love relationships and playtime with sex buddies.

★ You can be honest and still be discreet. "No, I'm not exclusive" or "Yes, I play with others" lets a partner know that you aren't cybermonogamous while maintaining the privacy of your harem.

Women adapt well to polyamory. We are used to having lots of close friends, building supportive networks and communities just through the natural way we live our lives. Set us free in an open space like the Internet, and those fears that drive us to possessiveness or jealousy drift away. It doesn't mean you're going to return to your offline partner and announce that you are now poly and he'd better get used to it, quick! But you might find yourself opening up to more ways to love him. And that's a good thing.

How to Manage a Harem Offline

HOTTEST!

"Parallel dating" is the latest hot phrase to describe . . . well . . . dating. It means you are seeing more than one person, and it implies that you are sleeping with at least two of them (although not necessarily at the same moment). It is not really polyamory in that you are not forming a group network of relationships so much as keeping your options open. I used to refer to it as "maintaining my harem"—but never to their faces.

Many, many books are available that delve deeply into this subject. This lesson looks at some ways you can use technology to keep up with this busy, if exhilarating, lifestyle.

★ Dedicate yourself to keeping your private "date calendar" current. If you use Google tools, you can create calendar entries from your email as long as the email contains enough hints for the application to pick up, like a date and time.

★ If you create custom playlists to listen to when you're with each partner, don't name the playlists by the person's name. It's important that each one know you aren't dating anyone exclusively, but you don't have to rub anyone's nose in it.

★ Conversely, when you add new lovers to your IM contact list, consider renaming them from their handles to their names, or at least adding their first name to the handle. This helps avoid slip-ups like calling out the wrong name when the flirting gets hot.

★ Mention early on in your email or IM conversations that you aren't looking for anything exclusive at this time; many women put a note about this in their dating profiles to turn away men who feel strongly about not sharing.

★ Hang out in alternative dating sites that cater to swingers and sexually open adults if you are looking for sex and polydating. These people will be more sanguine about your requirements than the innocent members of Match.com.

★ Follow the etiquette: Don't answer calls or texts from one date when you're out with another; don't tell Lover 1 all about the great time you had last weekend with Lover 2; don't play them off each other or passively aggressively foster competition among the group; don't keep all their toothbrushes in one mug on the bathroom counter. Discretion is not dishonesty.

How to Have Sex in Space

 HOT!

Do you think you'll have the opportunity to have sex in space in your lifetime? If not, the limitations are probably financial, not physical. George and Loretta Whitesides have already booked their space-going honeymoon, for 2009 or soon after. (If that sounds good to you, check spacelove.org for more information.)

Sex in space will require us to adapt to new ways of moving, touching, and getting intimate. We'll be dealing with motion sickness, and if we're in zero gravity, we'll have a fluids issue to contend with—perhaps the first "official" lovemaking will be by fully suited partners using sophisticated teledildonics systems!

Virgin Galactic (http://virgingalactic.com) is already taking reservations for space flights, while Bigelow Aerospace is rumored to be thinking about building a space hotel in Earth orbit (in which people will have sex). So it's not too soon to start planning.

> *Wherever we go in space, people will bring their humanity with them. We're not going to change so much as adapt physically to wherever we are living. We will still have our feelings, our sex drives, our drive to survive and reproduce.*
>
> —Laura Woodmansee, author, *Sex in Space*

LEARN TO CHOREOGRAPH

Sex without gravity might require Velcro or bondage tape to keep you from floating apart from one another. (Fun!)

BRING A TOWEL

People tend to sweat more in low gravity than in Earth normal. Don't forget to fasten the towel to yourself.

TALK

Communication becomes hugely important, because mechanics will be limited. As with sex in cyberspace, our brains will be called upon to provide most of the stimulation.

BANK EGGS AND SPERM

The radiation in space does quite a number on our reproductive ingredients. You will need to use birth control while you're up there, however. And just in case, save some eggs and sperm at home, in case you decide to have children after your return to Earth.

ENJOY THE VIEW

Part of the thrill of sex in space is the closeness you feel to your partner as you stand and gaze out at the Earth. The two of you are so small, and yet here you are standing on the border of the next frontier. You might experience an awe so profound you will remember it as the best sex of your life—even if you never even kissed.

How to Meet Your
Online Lover in Person

HOTTEST!

In magazine and TV reports about Internet dating, reporters are often so wide-eyed and incredulous that people meet online. Why this is considered crazy, when the whole point of the Internet is to connect people of like interests or goals, is beyond me.

The basics safety guidelines of meeting an online lover in person for the first time are the same as those I'm sure you'd follow on any first date: Tell someone where you'll be and when, arrange to check in by phone at a certain time, get your date's full name and contact information, and avail yourself of some Google searches before agreeing to meet (and make sure to meet in a public place).

But there's more. Meeting an online lover in person carries with it a heady mix of anticipation, desire, and expectation—balanced against your intellectual understanding that things might not work out as you hope.

One advantage of meeting online is that you can set aside anxieties about your bodies and concentrate on a mental and emotional connection. As those bonds develop, you probably exchanged pictures; you might have used webcams.

If you haven't done that, or if your lover has managed to be dishonest without ever once triggering a red flag for you (and be honest with yourself here—have you stifled doubts?), that first meeting can end in disappointment and sorrow.

But.

There's nothing like the first sight of each other, taking in the extra weight, the scar, the bald patch—whatever it is you and your lover worry about—and realizing that the connection between you is as strong as ever.

Your erotic imaginations are perfectly matched. Your memories of uninhibited cybersex, of the times when you went further in words than you have gone in person with a new lover, your months of "If I were there" and "If only I could touch you, taste you, breathe you" suddenly flooding your heart. And now you can touch, taste, and breathe each other—but now you're bodies, not just words.

One strategy I've used is to kiss even before we speak. Some folks feel awkward and tongue-tied when they first see each other, and some feel their stomach sink as they realize that "in the mind" was better than "in the flesh." But if you kiss, and put all that passion and connection and love you developed online into that kiss, the ice melts as desire flares between you. And if desire doesn't flare immediately, you've at least followed through on your agreement, and now you can get down to the business of getting to know each other's endearing and irritating quirks. I've known sexual attraction to build slowly over five or six hours (or three days) after I thought the online sizzle had turned to offline fizzle. I wouldn't be too quick to dismiss the meeting as a mistake if I were you.

When I first met Rich (not his real name) after a year and a half of love online and by phone, we couldn't speak. Our hearts were in our throats. We

MEETING KIT

★ Safer sex supplies: Condoms, dental dams, lube, arnica (in case you get delightful bruises you don't want to bring home)

★ Toys or other props that have special meaning for the two of you

★ The addresses and phone numbers of alternate lodgings in case you need to get to a safe place quick

★ Pajamas, toothbrush, clean underwear

★ Enough cash for cab fare if you need to leave in a hurry

★ A credit or debit card with enough room on it to get yourself out of there in the event of an emergency or a threat to your personal safety

★ Phone numbers of local friends, or friends of friends

★ Objects you've wanted to show each other: photo albums, figurines, clothing, fetishwear

★ Presents!

kissed, and I almost came right there. I don't even remember getting from the airport to the car, except that I floated rather than walked, and he took all my luggage.

But I do remember him pulling off the freeway several times when we could not contain ourselves another minute, trying to climb inside each other by lips and tongues alone. The two-hour drive from the airport to his small town took us three hours; ten minutes after getting there, we were wrapped around each other like teenagers at a drive-in; and our eagerness for each other grew, rather than faded, for the rest of the weeklong visit.

When I first arranged to meet Dave (not his real name) in person, I broke several of the rules. We met in a public place (the airport) but I had arranged to stay at his house while on a business trip even though I had not done nearly enough background research on him ahead of time. In that first moment of seeing him, all the horror stories flashed through my head. Was I about to be abducted and date raped? Would he give me his phone number now, at this late date, to give to my friend and my sister? What if he had a jealous partner and she broke into the apartment in the middle of the night with a machete? Everything turned out fine, and we were lovers and are still friends, and who knows what might happen for us in the future? But I've never gone into a meeting that blind since.

How to Have Cybersex

HOTTEST!

The old joke about typing one-handed doesn't cover the half of it. Entire books have been written on this subject, and although many of the other lessons in this book touch on important aspects of cybersex, in this lesson, the focus is on the mechanics of it all.

★ Play with language. I don't care if you're on webcam and have 3D avatars to boot—language is the foundation of cybersex, and language is the bridge between your minds, hearts, and bodies. Use words that shock and awaken; use imagery drawn from the erotic, the pornographic, and the innocuous. Weaving literary metaphor with raunchy sex talk keeps you both engaged.

★ Don't disappear halfway through. You wouldn't in real life, and you shouldn't in cybersex. If you think you will be interrupted, stick with flirting and save the cybersex for another day.

★ Select a handle you can stand to read and hear on a regular basis in a sexual context. "HotMama" will serve you better than "JakesMom," for example.

★ Take your time. You could get off by yourself in 10 minutes or less, so why bother with cyber if that's your only goal? Cybersex is as much about the story the two (or three, or four, or . . .) of you invent as it is about masturbation.

★ Don't be self-conscious or worried about your spelling or writing. As long as you say what you're imagining, you'll do fine.

★ Learn the power of "Mmmm"—a cybersex essential. Use it when you can't think of anything to say but it's your turn to type, when your lover says something so arousing you need to stop typing for a moment but need to show you're still there, and when the other is in the middle of writing an elaborate setup and needs a response but not help from you.

★ Another cybersex must: "a;kldfj;aj." No one expects you to type sensibly through an orgasm, but banging one hand on the keys lets him know that you're still with him, and what's more, that he's brought you to this moment. (This works both ways—if he's suddenly bellowing "AKL;DQADAJ BLK;JFDAKLJ;DF ;DFKJL;F" at you, you know you're da bomb.)

Part VII:

Identity

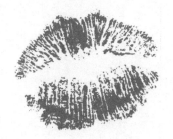

"One great thing about Internet culture is that you can be whoever you want to be and find out what it's like to present as a different gender, orientation, age, identity."

"The problem with the Internet is no one is who they appear to be."

At first glance, these statements appear to contradict each other. But you know what? After about a decade and a half online, I can tell you this: They're both true. And I'm not sure the second one is a problem.

I can't think of a single example of a venue in which you see all the facets of a person. We bring different aspects of ourselves to the forefront when at work, at church, at book clubs, at sex parties, at a friend's baby shower, on a singles' nature hike. Our parents see us one way, our lovers another, our bosses another.

I don't see why that should be any different online. I think when we say that everyone lies on the Internet, we are confusing two activities. For many women, exploring our identity through the sexy side of the Internet means unleashing fantasies or testing what it would be like to be "someone else"— someone we wonder if we could be "for reals." These are facets of ourselves we've buried or had to rein in because we think they're too wild or inappropriate for our offline lives.

Then there's the despicable practice of using an online identity to cause deliberate harm to another person, to manipulate people into unhealthy situations, to boost one's own ego and sense of empowerment by trampling on the hearts of others. This is the dark side of online identity (although this behavior is not limited to the Internet).

This section highlights a few of the less obvious forms of identity exploration—clones, alternate species, and (gasp!) being yourself. The Internet offers an incredible opportunity to unleash your imagination and discover more about your sexual self. You will probably find that once you open your personal Pandora's box, you won't be able to squish everything back in and lock the lid; and that this freedom will inspire and enhance your sex life hereafter.

How to Deal with Questions About Your Offline Identity

 HOT!

One thing that happens when you start to get close to people online is they start asking you about your offline life. If you're not ready to give that information out, sometimes things can get a little tense. Your lover might feel you don't trust him, or you might feel sorely tempted to divulge, but something you can't quite identify is holding you back.

Listen to that feeling. Once you've said it, you can't take it back.

I've always been polite and direct about this sort of thing. "I'm not comfortable giving that kind of information out" and "I prefer to keep my offline life private for now, but thank you for your interest" have both worked for me in the past.

Most folks are sensitive to issues of privacy and safety, particularly in adult communities, and so most folks will understand your hesitation. Because online intimacy happens so fast, it's easy to say too much too soon and regret it later. An online lover who pesters you for identifying information after you have explained that you're not comfortable or not ready for sharing that does not deserve to be your lover. They obviously don't have your best interests at heart if they're trying to browbeat or manipulate you into something you don't want to do.

Exchanging your legal identities with an online love is akin to a marriage. It's a level of commitment reserved for the most stable relationships, where you're taking things offline, at least as far as telephones and PO Boxes. Your street address is not something to hand out casually, because it can so easily be used against you by a stalker or an impersonator. Even though it's more likely your online lover will just say "cool" and have a fun time looking at your roof on Google Earth, you don't lose anything by waiting until after you've met in person to give out your home address.

That doesn't mean you can't both open a mailbox somewhere for exchanging tangible items! It's fun to send each other things like cookies, panties, books, DVDs, candles, shoes. Having an object you can stroke and smell and taste while you connect in virtual spaces brings you yet another notch closer together.

And so does sharing details about the rest of your life. I don't mind giving my name out after I develop trust with someone. I know this puts me at some risk of being found; that's a risk I'm willing to take. (I have a large dog and share a yard with my neighbors' two pit bulls, who often come into my house for playdates, so I'm not as worried as I might have been back when my only protector was a guinea pig.)

As with everything else in online relationships, honest communication serves you best. But that doesn't mean revealing details you aren't ready to share. You are not obligated to give out personal information, even if your lover has already shared such details with you.

And when that online lover becomes an offline partner too? If you meet in person and the love and trust only intensifies, that's when to make a fun ritual out of exchanging further details like full names and driver's license pictures.

How to Use Your Clone
(When You Get One)

 HOT!

Pet-cloning is already commercially available, for less money than you might think. So who knows how long it will be before we can clone ourselves, and *really* double our pleasure?

These are just a few examples of the fun to come. And as an added bonus, they give you some great counterpoints the next time someone rants about the evils of cloning. These tips outline some of the many ways you can use a clone.

★ Easily provide a third in a ménage à trois (or the ninth in a *neuftet,* as the case may be, or depending on how many clones you have.)

★ Send your double to traffic school, the DMV, or the post office while you send come-hither glances to scandalously too-young-for-you hotties on the beach.

★ Be S *and* M, at the same time.

★ Stay home reading a great novel while your clone wires up on a dozen first dates at Starbucks, screening online dating prospects.

★ Find out whether those jeans do indeed flatter your butt.

★ Practice new sexual positions before you spring them on your lover.

★ Be your own videographer.

★ Have cybersex and still be able to type with at least two hands.

★ Find out what you really look like during orgasm.

★ Be your spouse's wife *and* mistress.

★ Publish a clone fetish website and get rich off the membership dues.

★ Scratch where it itches.

How to Be Yourself Online

 HOT!

We often think of the Internet as a place where people can try on different lives, and many of the lessons in this section show the benefits of experimenting with aspects of your identity.

Still, I believe that no matter who you choose to be online, you are still yourself. Being on the Internet does not make you a different person. It *can* open your eyes to entirely new facets of yourself, though. I know more than one person whose online explorations were the final step in decisions like leaving a marriage, starting a new career, and even getting transgender surgery. Others might interpret this as "You went online, and now you're someone else." But in my experience, it's been more like, "The self you never showed finally had a chance to shine, and you chose to integrate that part of you more fully into your life."

Being yourself online is practical. For one thing, it's easier to sustain than an alter ego. If you start forming strong love relationships with other people and talking about meeting in person someday, you don't have to have a Long Conversation about who you "really" are. I know of one woman who went online as a gay man and fell in love; years into the relationship, she came clean; they still love one another, but the relationship had to go through some pretty incredible discussions and decisions and hard work to reach its balance point.

When you are your full self online, you feel more secure that the relationships you make are genuine, based on who you are, not just on one aspect of yourself that you choose to show. You still need to go through the work of finding out whether the other person is being fully themselves if you plan to meet in person.

Often, we start out with an alter ego and think we're being someone very different—and then we discover that we actually *are* that person too. At that point, embracing and integrating all the aspects of ourselves leads to deeper, more intimate relationships on many levels.

See Part VIII for tips on keeping yourself safe online. Being your real, true, honest self does not extend to handing out your address, the name of your company, or your favorite private hiking trail.

Here are ways to be yourself while still keeping yourself safe.

★ Be honest about your age, marital status, children, dreams, and aspirations.

★ If you've been sharing things with an online lover you have never told anyone else, make sure to also share things everyone already knows about you. Otherwise, your lover will get to know only one side of you, the deep and personal, and not have any context for the rest of you. And why wouldn't you want them to know that funny story of how you ran away from home when you were six, or how you still haven't gotten over that humiliating spelling bee in high school? It's all part of being yourself.

★ If you are in an offline relationship and you find yourself only sharing the sad stuff about it, but you actually like the person you're with, share the good stuff too. (If you don't like the person you're with, you might reconsider your decision to be with that person.) Again, only showing part of the truth deprives your online lover of getting to know your full self.

★ Take responsibility for revealing what you are feeling. If you have a twinge of sadness, laughter, jealousy, fear, hunger—say so. As intimate and deep as online connections can be—and as often as we seem to read each other's minds and hearts with uncanny accuracy—that communication level breaks down under stress or fatigue, and it's unfair to expect anyone to know your every nuance if you don't share it. And share in a complete and honest manner, like "I just felt a twinge of envy just now, but I'm also really happy for you" or "I just welled up with tears, that was so beautiful, thank you."

★ Interactive chat can be stream-of-consciousness in both thought and format. (Say *this* the next time someone starts rhapsodizing about James Joyce's literary style: He was just ahead of his time, telling a story as if he were in a chat room.) And when you are involved as your true self without the shield of a persona, you sometimes take things more personally than your lover intended. Don't judge every word or phrase beyond its moment of context. We're human, we have flaws, and we suffer miscommunication. We are more open to growth when we accept that we may be misunderstood, and we may misunderstand our partner's words.

★ Take time to explain your personal slang and shorthand. Besides helping you communicate better, new conversations can arise from your explanations of the history of the words that you use.

How to Find Support to Come Out as Whoever You Are, Sexually

 HOT!

Many of us question our sexuality at some point in our lives. An extended period of no sex drive might leave you wondering whether you are actually asexual. A sudden crush on a girl might make you wonder whether you are lesbian or bisexual, or whether you're just jumping on the "bi is cool" bandwagon to spice up your love life. A sense of gender dysphoria—discomfort with your assigned gender—might start to feel like it's too much to bear without help. And if you've always surrounded yourself with women and preferred female lovers, it can be terribly disconcerting to find yourself developing romantic feelings for a guy online!

Or quite possibly your online play has revealed your desire for pain, or bondage, or threesomes, or some other "kink" you are not sure your partner will understand or want to take part in.

The Internet has taught us that whatever we are, someone else is too. And however bad we've got it, someone else has it worse—and someone else has been there ahead of us and smoothed the path.

Refer to "How to Find an Adult Community with Nice, Smart People In It" on page 58 for tips on how to evaluate and enter a supportive environment. Meanwhile, these sites will help you find people to connect with as you enter this part of your journey. Note that this is only a tiny portion of the communities available to you online; I couldn't possibly list them all.

ASEXUAL VISIBILITY AND EDUCATION NETWORK

The Asexual Visibility and Education Network (AVEN) supports people who do not experience sexual attraction. "Unlike celibacy, which is a choice, asexuality is a sexual orientation," says the home page. "Asexual people have the same emotional needs as everybody else and are just as capable of forming intimate relationships." Given the highly sexualized nature of our popular media, asexual people can feel ostracized and "broken." If that's you or someone you know, AVEN is an excellent place to learn more and talk with others who feel the same way. See www.asexuality.org.

LESBIAN WORLDS

The Lesbian Worlds' Coming Out site (www.lesbianworlds.com/out) offers women a place to tell their stories, even if they can't come out anywhere else due to political, family, or work pressures.

TG FORUM

The TG Forum offers an extensive resource list for people seeking more information about transgenderism. It also hosts personal ads for members. See http://tgforum.com.

SECOND LIFE

The virtual world of Second Life is chock-full of groups exploring various forms of sexuality, with regular discussions about love and sexuality hosted by different people and groups. Search the Events and Groups listings for keywords related to what you're exploring and don't be shy about contacting the hosts for more information. See http://secondlife.com.

How to Be Bisexual
on the Internet

HOTTEST!

If you're already bisexual, you can skip this lesson. These tips are for those who are questioning, experimenting, or exploring.

It has always seemed to me that the part of cybersex that attracts the most criticism—the absence of touch—is the part that gives it such potential to deepen our understanding of sex. It's no bad thing to set aside our bodies once in awhile and just be people, no matter what our plumbing looks like.

Many people who aren't otherwise bisexual happily flirt and cyber with any gender online. After all, unless you plan to meet your partners in person for sex and you know you're not interested in physical same- or hetero-sex (and are you sure about that?), why should it matter? The Internet offers a perfect, private place to experiment without much risk.

★ It's okay to explain that you are only bi online.

★ The "woman" you are cybering with might be a man on the other side of the keyboard. So what? If you're having fun, have fun. You'll meet a nice girl some other time.

★ Play with language and let your imagination roam. If you've never made love with a woman before, you have a whole different topography to deal with now.

★ In a public room, women will often flirt and "make out" with each other to enhance the sexual ambience, but then wind down before it turns into "sex" (and believe me, those lines blur more and more every year).

★ If you start playing with a woman with the intention of turning on the men watching, it's not uncommon for your focus to shift. The first time I did this, I was amazed to find my body responding and my interest sharpening. I forgot about our audience and got into our session, even though I'd never even kissed a woman before.

How to Deal If You Share Your Name with a Porn Star

 HOT!

Gina Lynn. Violet Blue. Doug Jefferies. All three of these are friends of mine who are not porn stars. And yet if you—or a prospective employer—Google any of these names, the results will show an interesting blend of their own activities and porn star biographies.

As our online reputations become more central to our lives, what is associated with our names takes on great significance in job searches, credit applications, and even dating. Sometimes I wonder whether, instead of an "Objective" as the first line of a resume, we should be putting a note about who we are and aren't: "Identity: Gina Lynn—the writer, not the porn star."

Most recruiters won't expect a currently performing porn star to apply for a job in information technology or customer service, even though many porn actresses have skills and training other than on-camera sex. Even so, you don't want people making assumptions (and developing expectations) about who you are based on what other people are doing under your name.

A porn star is not going to change her brand simply because you are applying for a teaching credential and your name really is Ginger von Cream. Therefore it is up to you to know whether your name has been co-opted, so you can be prepared to respond to questions about it.

The problem gets stickier when you have an online presence of your own. Violet Blue, the nonporn star, has a tremendously popular website in which she writes about sex. She is a columnist, a blogger, a best-selling author, a model, and above all, a sex educator. Thus, searching for her online brings up links to her amazing oeuvre—and to a porn star's activities.

One adult event confused the two and ran the wrong picture in its flyers. The porn star has been quoted expressing opinions diametrically opposed to the writer's. Violet combats the confusion by remaining proactive about her identity and posting "I am not a porn performer" right up there on her home page.

If you're a teacher or a pediatrician or in some other child-related profession, be especially vigilant about what shows up next to "your" name online. By now, we should understand that we can't believe everything we read online, and we should give each other the benefit of the doubt.

If your name is your brand, get an attorney, and file all the appropriate legal documents on it: trademarks, service marks, whatever is appropriate to your business. Learn how to use keywords, tags, titles, and other metadata on your website to create a distinct and specific description of your presence for major search engines.

You can also consider using a different name or brand if you find that your porn star twin is already established and has some longevity. When I first started writing "Sex Drive" in 2003, my byline was Gina Lynn. But when Gina Lynn

the adult actress filed a trademark on the name, I changed my byline to Regina
Lynn to help eliminate the confusion. It wasn't a legal necessity, but it did help
people tell us apart.

The important thing is to remain aware of who else comes up in a Google
search for your name. And then be as proactive as you need to be to manage
your identity.

How to Explore
Other Sentient Species

 HOTTER!

Paranormal is one of the most popular subgenres in romantic and erotic fiction. Vampires and werewolves abound, with time travelers and faeries at a close second.

Sex lends itself so well to fantasy that it sometimes surprises me how often our online activity reflects regular ole sex, bound by the laws of physics and our own human bodies.

Online spaces give us an outlet for our most creative storytelling. In cybersex, you can be animals, aliens, ghosts, historical figures, and famous fictional characters. You can make love in a spaceship, a planetary prison colony, or a dragon's cave.

I have made love as a wolf—a true one, not a werewolf—and discovered a whole new language, one that is sensual and raw and physical and doesn't use human words. Animal sex, for us anyway, is all actions and body language and species-appropriate vocalizations.

Mixing and matching among species encourages a mindset open to adaptation and connection. Just how would a twelve-inch pixie have sex with a seven-foot elf? Would a wild mustang stallion really have a chance at that Olympic-level dressage mare through her security fencing and reinforced stall doors?

Love always finds a way.

★ Virtual worlds are tailor-made for interspecies romance due to their rich visual environment. Any Second Life club event is likely to have nonhuman creatures in attendance, and you can search for fantasy-themed areas to increase your chances of courting an elf or faerie or god or goddess. Or wend your way to a spaceport; if you don't find one, you can always build one. (That's the nature of 3D—what was here today may not be there tomorrow, but something else will be.)

★ If you've heard of "Furries," you know there is already a strong community of people online who role-play as animals, both biological and mythological. What you might not realize is this is a diverse and publicity-shy bunch who really hate to be gawked at and held up as the example of the crazy things people do online. Much of the time, Furries aren't even involved in sexual activity—they're just enjoying being their animal selves. So if this fantasy appeals to you, approach the community with humility and respect, showing that you are serious about the play and not there to ridicule anyone. That means having an avatar ready if you're in a 3D world, or at least asking someone to help you create an appropriate avatar, and being patient with the time and energy it takes to become welcomed into the pack. Or flock. Or whatever.

★ You can always ease into animal or other nonhuman roles with your current partner. They might feel too silly or self-conscious to play with it offline at first, but slip easily into the fantasy over instant message, starting with some gentle in-character flirting and then taking it wherever y'all decide to take it.

★ A text chat room can also provide a venue for species role-play, especially if you're a regular and it's a fun, creative group. Show up one day and instead of your usual handle, give yourself an animal name and start acting like that animal, dropping enough clues that your friends figure out that it's you (or at least that it's someone they know).

How to Be a Man Online

HOTTER!

Why be a man? Maybe you're tired of the constant barrage of "A/S/L" (age/sex/location) private messages, or maybe you want to flirt from the other team's bench. Perhaps there's a desire to wield a digital penis. It doesn't really matter why, but it does matter whether you can actually pull it off convincingly.

Let me plant my tongue firmly in my cheek and give you some tips on masquerading as a man online. These will help you ensure that women don't fall so in love with you that they leave their families and move across the world to stalk you.

★ Think like a man before you even decide on a screen name. Most men don't bother to hide their intentions (especially in an anonymous online situation), but some will tease you with wordplay until you beg them to rip your clothes off. So what kind of man do you want to be? Are you "SexManiac10Inches" or "LookingForLoveInUniquePlaces"?

★ Cut the flowery language. Men who "tenderly lick a steaming trail along the flesh of your inner thigh" are likely professional writers on a break, and men who "lovingly massage the wonderful shape of your tits" are unconvincing. It's true, there are men who can fire your romantic soul with passionate prose, but unless you want the woman falling head over heels for your online persona, stick to the basics. "Rubbing your breasts. Mmm yeah" is a good example.

★ Be aggressive. You are no longer the hen watching the mating dance; you're now the cock, proudly displaying your plumage. Remember, many women are accustomed to these aggressive rituals, and you're competing with real men accustomed to performing them. Get in there and shake it!

★ Be persistent. No means no, but "Well . . ." can mean "I need to see more." Show her more, and then show her even more for good measure. If she's still unimpressed, move on without getting discouraged. It's good practice, and with practice comes success.

★ Have fun! You love a man who has a good sense of humor and can show you a good time, right? Put on the robe and wizard hat and have a few laughs— but don't forget to take them off in the heat of passion.

Okay, okay, maybe you want to try being a man online to learn something about yourself, to experience first-hand the assumptions we make in our society based on gender or to practice making love to women. In that case, you can sprinkle your conversation with "guy slang" and use "male words" for female body parts and functions. Pattern yourself on a man you know and borrow his favorite movies, cars, and sports.

If you're just playing, don't toy with others' hearts. If someone, male or female, seems to be falling for you, discourage them.

But you don't have to ruin the fantasy with the truth. You're a man now. Cowboy up and accept it.

How to Reveal Yourself
(and How to Know When It's Time)

HOTTER!

Many people reach a point in an online relationship when they realize they want to reveal themselves utterly to another person. This may be because you've fallen in love and have started to talk about meeting in person. Or it might just be that the other person trusted you with his mother's maiden name and his social security number, and you want to reciprocate with your legal first name.

Yet if you look around, you'll find happy couples who met this way—in chat rooms, in forums, in games, in online dating profiles. Certainly before they met in person, they had enough information about each other's identity to Google one another, and they felt comfortable with what they found.

It's hard to say when the "right time" is. As with most relationships, you'll need to make your decisions based on what works for the two of you and what you feel is right.

Here are some general tips for when to exchange full names.

In many cultural myths and legends, names have special significance. One common theme is that knowing a person's "true name" gives you power over him or her. Think of what happened to Rumpelstiltskin. And did you notice how careful Harry Potter's mentors were about not using the real name of You Know Who, lest he feel it and turn his attention to them?

In today's data-driven world, names do confer power. Look at the difference in how people respond to you when you enter a chat room or virtual world as "LoveBeALady" versus "Horneyslut19" versus "David." If you've tried online dating, notice how much weight you placed on the person's chosen display name. I would take "LAstud" less seriously than "ChefonaQuest," as the former indicates frat boy bragging (a sure sign of insecurity and immaturity) while the latter hints at the person's passion and skill.

Sharing your name online is a sign that you trust the other person won't use it against you—and you should receive other people's names with the respect and dignity the gift deserves.

★ You start talking about meeting in person and are already researching airfares and hotels.

★ You are talking frankly about your job, your life, your kids, your friends, and your hobbies, and only then realize that you've been perfectly comfortable doing so all along.

★ You realize you feel closer to this person than almost anyone else in your life, and you would like to hear them whisper your name rather than your handle.

As for how to do it: Some people make it a ceremony and plan a special date in which they gift their names to one another. Others simply find themselves saying "by the way, my name is . . ." in the course of the conversation.

Then there's what happened to me with one of my chat buddies years ago. He spent almost two weeks saying he wanted to tell me his full name, and then backing off. It was a huge deal for him, and certainly he put much more weight on it than I did. I'd already given him my full name and my phone number, so it's not like we weren't close. I was patient and didn't push and in truth I'd stopped caring, and then one day he called me on the phone and spent 10 or 15 minutes dithering before he blurted it out.

At which point I promptly forgot it. To this day, I have only vaguest idea that it might have started with "Mc."

Once you exchange names, search for each other like crazy, digging up old high school photos or blog posts or book reviews you posted to Amazon ten years ago. This is where you reveal yourself as a person with a past—and perhaps as a person with some "splainin" to do. (It's a good idea to Google yourself beforehand so you know what your lover is going to see.)

Part VIII:

Safety

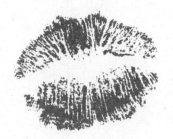

Pedophiles! Infidelity! Perverts!

Somehow, we've developed a big cultural fear about the Internet. However, we do need to take some precautions to keep ourselves safe online, just like we do in any other part of our lives. Much has been written about how to meet people offline in safe and sane ways—the same strategies that sex workers have used for ages—and you can find those tips at any online dating site.

This section introduces some of the basic principles of safer sex and safer computing. However, because this is the one topic every other author covers in gleeful detail, I've chosen not to focus on it too much in this book. Think ahead, use common sense—and have fun.

How to Obscure
Your Digital Trail

 HOT!

It's impossible to hide yourself totally and still play online.
However, if you follow some basic guidelines, you can minimize the risk of
being caught in compromising positions.

Note that this is only the easy, basic stuff. If you're paranoid, you will want
to buy some books about encryption, data management, and privacy.

★ Create email and message chat accounts specifically for use in adult
communities, and use these accounts only for this purpose, so you don't mix
friend-and-family mail with cybersex mail.

★ Use a pseudonym when you register for any community, and make it a
gender-neutral first name and a surname that can pass for a first name.
Names like Cameron Alexander, Terry Casey, Madison Stone, will confound
database search engines and make cross-references that much harder. If early
trust develops in an online relationship, you can always reveal that your
cyber name is not your real name, while reserving your true identity as a
surprise for a special occasion.

★ Use an Internet browser that allows you to clear caches and cookies. By clearing these out from the browser's storage, it will be harder to track your digital trail from your web browser. Mozilla's Firefox web browser warns if it suspects a website is a forgery (a "phishing" site), protects from spyware, and most importantly, clears the cache (a history of where you've been) with just one click. If you use the Firefox browser, you can set it to clear private data such as browser history, cookies, and form information every time you close it. Go to Tools > Options > Privacy and check "Always clear my private data when I close Firefox." Click the Settings button to select which data to clear and which to keep.

★ Don't use your work computer for things you don't want your boss, the entire IT team, or the CEO to know. Even a company-owned BlackBerry-like wireless device will record logs.

★ Shop online for playthings with a one-time-use credit card number. PayPal (www.paypal.com) offers a virtual debit card that generates a different "account number" for every transaction. Your real credit card number is not shared all over the Internet, and the merchant never knows that this is a proxy credit card number.

★ If you feel the need for an extra tier of Internet privacy, consider a service like http://anonymizer.com, http://proxyking.net, or http://proxyguy.com. These place a layer of confidentiality between you and the websites you visit, or the email that you send.

How to Protect Yourself from Online Stalkers

 HOT!

Anywhere you get a group of people together, you're going to have two things: sexual tension (yay!) and creepy bastards (boo!).

Cyberstalking is the use of the Internet, email, or other electronic communications to stalk and harass another person. Just like technology makes it easier for us to connect with more hearts, it also makes it easier for these numbskulls to obsess about you and let you know it, without giving you a positive ID to hand to the police.

E-stalkers can manipulate third parties to harass or threaten you. They can impersonate you and post inflammatory messages in your name, or flame you across blogs and message boards. If a stalker gets hold of your name, address, or other personal information, the harassment can continue offline as well.

I've never been stalked, although I've had one or two people refuse to take no for an answer and continue to IM or email me, changing their accounts after I blocked them. They eventually got bored and stopped hounding me; my policy of ignoring such nonsense worked in those cases. Unfortunately, it doesn't always work.

IF YOU'RE A TARGET

If despite your efforts to prevent it, you find yourself the target of a cyberstalker, here are some strategies to follow to get them off your back.

Ask once, and only once, that all communication or contact be stopped. Make it crystal clear that this is unwanted contact.

Do not get into a dialogue or series of exchanges with the stalker. Be firm. It is not your job to soothe egos.

Save all digital files for evidence. Do not edit or alter them in any way. Also, keep a record of your interactions with digital service providers or law enforcement officials. Report any threat of violence to law enforcement.

Consider changing your email, Internet, and phone service providers. If the cyberstalking extends to your workplace, inform your employer, and ask for any resources to help stop the harassment at work.

Many jurisdictions have cyberstalking laws. Contact your local law enforcement and prosecutor's office for information.

The National Center for Victims of Crime maintains a Stalking Resource at www.ncvc.org/src. You can also visit http://wiredsafety.org for information about cyber abuse.

Harassment is harassment, regardless of where or how it takes place. If it is distressing you enough to interfere with your daily life, health, or work, report it to the police like you would any other harassment.

Here are some tips to help you avoid the situation, and how to address it if it occurs.

★ Do not share personal information in virtual spaces anywhere online, including in email, forums, and role-playing games.

★ Do not use your real name or nickname as your screen name. Create a name that is gender and age neutral.

★ Make sure that your ISP and virtual space and social websites have an acceptable use policy that prohibits cyberstalking. Check this before you sign up—every site has a User Agreement or Terms of Service to read as part of the registration. Skip it at your peril.

★ If your service provider fails to respond to your complaints, consider switching to a more responsive provider. Check www.broadbandreports.com for ISP user recommendations and reviews.

★ Use an Internet search engine like Google to check your real name for your current presence on the Internet. Many of our Big Life Moments become matters of public record. Marriages, divorces, probate, real estate—not to mention that infamous spring break. This will give you an idea of what's already out there so you can minimize the impact of a cybercreep spreading lies about you later.

How to Find
the Right Condoms

HOTTER!

The condom may be the most ubiquitous example of applied technology addressing a need in human sexuality. However, if you've been monogamous or celibate for ten, fifteen, or twenty years, you might not realize just how far we've come in prophylactic technology since you last had to pay attention.

Condoms are the specialized athletic sportswear of the new millennium. There are more styles of condom than balloons in a circus. The range addresses a variety of user needs: size, sensitivity, lubrication, durability, taste, aesthetics, and allergies.

It's easier to use (or go back to using, *sigh*) condoms when we find the brands and styles that are the most comfortable and the least interruptive for us—and then use them consistently and well. If you try to see condoms as a standard, nonnegotiable part of sex rather than a huge imposition, you'll be playing safe while having more fun. (And if you think it's an imposition, imagine the inconvenience of being HIV positive.)

MATERIALS

Condoms come in three main materials: latex, polyurethane, and lambskin. Lambskin only protects against pregnancy, though, not sexually transmitted

---

NO ON NONOXYNOL-9

For years, nonoxynol-9 was a popular spermicidal lubricant and was even touted as a microbicide in the fight against sexually transmitted infections. It's now widely held that nonoxynol-9 can cause membrane irritation and actually increase the risk of sexually transmitted infections due to small abrasions in the vagina through which a virus can pass.

---

infections. Latex is the most common choice; polyurethane is popular with those who are sensitive or allergic to latex.

SIZES

Because no two penises are alike in size, shape, or owner skill, condoms are increasingly made in various sizes and head styles. If you have a regular partner who isn't a regular fit, try some of the sized condoms. Always go for reality (regular) over ego (jumbo extra large) for comfort and protection.

THICKNESS

Condoms can have thin or thick latex wall. Thinner walls are claimed to make the condom less noticeable, while thicker walls cut down on sensation to help a man last longer. Some "climax control" condoms actually use a small amount of benzocaine to slightly numb the penis.

FLAVOR

Latex will never be the flavor of the month at the local ice cream shop. But

CONDOM SHOPPING ONLINE

CONDOMDEPOT.COM

Since 1996, owner Kimberly Fidi has offered a confidential website with great service at a reasonable cost.

CONDOMANIA.COM

Condomania has retail store, mail order, and online divisions. The Condom Wizard is an online questionnaire that will guide you to the right condom for you, based on your responses.

UNDERCOVERCONDOMS.COM

This website offers an animated condom selector.

---

flavored condoms do make protected oral sex more fun. You can go for cooling mint, invigorating citrus, or tropical banana—it seems they come up with more flavors every year. Some brands offer a "warming" cinnamon or "tingling" peppermint, while others are more subtle, giving you just a hint of sweetness to alleviate the taste of latex. Condomania offers several sampler packs with a variety of brands and flavors, so don't be afraid to experiment.

SHAPES

Perhaps you're inspired by the shape of things to come. The contoured condoms with ribs, studs, and spiral twists can give you a little extra oomph that almost makes up for not being able to go skin-on-skin. On the other hand, you might find that the nubs and bumps irritate your delicate tissues, or that the "balloon-tipped" condoms bang uncomfortably into your cervix. It never hurts to have a regular condom nearby in case you need to do a quick wardrobe change when things heat up.

LUBE

Even lubricated condoms can "catch" at your (or his) delicate skin, and with all that friction, the loss of lubrication makes a condom prone to breakage. Have lube handy and a small spray bottle of water for rewetting as needed. Make sure to buy latex-compatible lube, though; oils and petroleum products will break down a latex condom and render it useless as protection.

TOYS

Condom makers have noticed that women are a lot less reluctant to talk about, review, and use toys as part of their everyday sexual experience. Condoms packaged with one-time-use vibrating rings combine protection with pleasure and also give you a nonthreatening way to introduce toys into partner sex.

FEMALE CONDOMS AND DENTAL DAMS

All the same considerations about materials apply to female condoms and dental dams. However, these are pretty much one-size-fits-most, and you don't have nearly the same range of choices as you do with male condoms. If it's your first time using these your best bet is to contact a knowledgeable staff person with your particular concerns.

How to Get Tested for Sexually Transmitted Infections from Home

HOT!

The best thing to do if you suspect you have contracted a sexually transmitted infection is to get to a doctor. Many STIs are curable if you catch and treat them early enough; herpes can't be cured yet, but it's not life-threatening, and modern treatments can make you much more comfortable.

But sometimes, for some reason, people can't or won't go to the clinic. Maybe they are worried that the news will leak, or maybe they contracted an STI while cheating and need to get diagnosed and treated before passing it on to their partner—who has not consented to this risk. A cheated-on partner already has enough to deal with when their lover cheats; adding an STI on top of that is not a loving thing to do.

COMPREHENSIVE TESTING WITH LAB WORK

At http://tstd.org and http://stdweb.com, you order the tests online and have them sent to your home or other safe place. These services can screen you for several STIs, including chlamydia, gonorrhea, syphilis, HIV, herpes, and

PROACTIVE AND POSITIVE

According to a 2002 survey published in the American Journal of Public Health, fewer than one-third of U.S. physicians included STI screening as part of a routine physical.

Being proactive in seeking assurance in our sexual health is an important component of positive sexuality. Be open and honest with your healthcare professional about your partners and practices, and don't let any doctor make you feel ashamed of it. If you're embarrassed to bring it up while naked and spread out with your feet in the stirrups, tell the nurse you need to see the doctor first, while you're still dressed, to address a concern before the exam.

Even when you're doing your best to practice safer sex, sometimes accidents happen, and if you go to the doctor, you've done the responsible thing. If your doctor doesn't help you feel comfortable, switch practitioners.

hepatitis B and C, and include a visit to a local lab. Given the nature of the service, your privacy is protected every step of the way.

You get a PIN so you can check your results online and even share them with your partner through an online interface.

AT-HOME COLLECTION

Home Access (http://homeaccess.com) and DirectDX (http://directdx.com) offer limited STI and other tests you can purchase online. You do the "lab work" at home and mail the test back, then await results.

RAPID TESTING KITS

First Diagnostic makes immediate-results tests for a number of STIs. Results are not quite as reliable as with the tests where you collect the appropriate fluid and send it in to a lab, and it is possible to have a false positive or a false negative. However, if you do a few tests about three weeks apart—to give your body time to create antibodies for the test to detect—you will have a pretty good idea of whether you've picked up a virus. See www.atfirstdiagnostic.com.

How to Cope When Your Video Sex Session Goes Public Without Your Permission

 HOT!

Our communications technologies allow for private text or images to be shared with thousands of people in a heartbeat. And once it's done, there's no going back. It's too late. It's been archived, pushed out on feeds, blogged—when it's out there, it's out there.

It's one thing when private material is disseminated by accident. But when a person decides to wield that power with malice, it really chaps my hide. Some people are just trying to find new ways to hurt others when the rest of us are trying to share the love. Mean people suck.

The impact of such unwanted publicity can graduate in scale from social embarrassment to job loss, family distress, and emotional crisis. (Unless you're a budding celebrity, in which case it means more record sales and more tabloid publicity.)

Even an innocuous photo or text message, altered by a harassing tech-geek, can cause harm. All it takes is a person with a grudge and good photo-editing skills to turn your simple bikini-on-the-beach vacation snapshot into a nude.

If you're in a profession where you work with children, such malice can have devastating consequences, if your employer decides to fire you "just in case."

These tips can help you cope if you're caught in a situation like this.

★ Don't give in to total, utter despair. This too shall pass. The blogosphere abounds with stories of people who got fired for things they wrote in their blogs who went on to bigger and better careers elsewhere.

★ Share pictures cautiously. I hate that this cuts into the fun, but until you trust someone with your entire life and know for sure it's not misplaced faith, keep your face out of the photos. (And if they break your heart later by breaking that trust? Ache, rage, and cry—but don't sink to the same lows. They'll get even worse than what they gave, eventually.)

★ If your chat buddy pushes you to put your face in a naughty picture, he's not the nice guy you thought he was. Nice guys understand our caution and appreciate what we're willing to share without pushing for images that could get us in trouble later.

★ Get ahead of the damage wave. Diffuse the shock by preparing your inner circle. Tell your trusted friends that you may be the target of Internet abuse if you become aware of such an incident.

★ Don't be ashamed of your activity. If the person who published your privates is trying to shame you, counter with the attitude that's it's not shameful to express love and lust. It is a perversion of trust to use intimate imagery without consent. Attempting to do mischief or harm by misusing intimate expressions places shame only on the abuser.

★ If your employer becomes involved, contact a knowledgeable attorney and examine your legal rights. Certain occupations may have established "moral" clauses in the employment conditions, particularly in professions in which adults work with youth and children. If you're a teacher, a youth group counselor, a pediatrician, or in a related career, the consequences of online sex play can hit you much harder than the rest of us. However, the good news is that as more and more of us are "outed" in our play, the impact lessens. Eventually teachers will have as much freedom as the rest of us, so hang in there!

★ You can try to contact the hosting website or Internet service provider to remove the offending files. That can take some time, but it's worth doing not just to get the files offline but to create a record of your attempts to remedy the problem. Even if someone else downloads the files and posts them on another site, making every effort to take them down works in your favor. Eventually the furor will die down and your efforts will pay off.

★ Several organizations have formed in recent years to help people manage their online reputations. They scour the web for mentions of their clients—everyone from CEOs to celebrities—and shape the digital trail to suit the client's goal. You can find a list of these services at http://jcwarner.com/reputation.

Sex-Tech Glossary

Cee

3D WORLD. See "Virtual World"

AUDIO-DRIVEN VIBRATOR. A vibrator that responds to an audio source, such as an iPod, a computer speaker, a DVD player, or your voice. The vibrations adjust in time to the music or pulse of sound.

BLUETOOTH. A communication method that allows electronic devices to talk to one another.

CHAT ROOM. A place where people gather online. Can be text-only, webcam, audio, 3D, but generally refers to text or video.

COMMUNITY. What forms when two or more people interact on a regular basis online. The foundation for the sexual revolution 2.0.

INTIMATE INTERFACE. The marketing term intended to replace "teledildonics," because the latter is too scary a word.

MMO. This stands for "massively multiplayer online" and is sometimes followed by "RPG" ("role-playing game") or "EG" ("erotic game"). *World of Warcraft* is the most famous current example, at press time.

ONLINE DATING. A database model for matchmaking in which you fill out a profile describing yourself and try to get connected with other people like you.

PLAYLIST. A collection of songs generally organized by a particular theme, such as "upbeat" or "sexy."

PORN. The backbone of internet commerce.

RPG. Role-playing game. An online video game in which many players participate and interact with one another. (By contrast, some games have only one real player, and all the other individuals are simply in-game characters.)

RSS FEED. A way to have content delivered to you so that you don't have to visit every website in search of information or entertainment.

SMS. See "Text Message."

SOCIAL NETWORKING. The same as online dating only people pretend they aren't interested in finding sex partners.

STREAM. Content that travels from somewhere else (the "server") to your computer (the "client") while you listen to or view it. You don't have to download the whole thing to your hard drive before you can enjoy it.

TELEDILDONICS. Any form of controlling a sexual or romantic device across a network, such as the Internet or a mobile phone network.

TEXT MESSAGE. A text missive sent over the mobile phone network, generally limited to a certain number of characters. Also known as SMS ("short message service").

VIRTUAL WORLD. Chat room meets virtual reality, where you create a digital representation of yourself and interact with other people through their digital representations (known as avatars). Also called 3D worlds. They are basically role-playing games without the "game" part. Second Life is the most current famous example, at press time.

WEB 2.0. Buzzword for the different ways in which the Internet is becoming more user-oriented, enabling users to organize, create, and contribute content and to interact with each other and with the content more easily than in the past.

About the Author

Regina Lynn is the "Sex Drive" columnist at Wired.com and the author of *The Sexual Revolution 2.0*. She won a Maggie award for Best Online Column from the Western Publications Association and was a finalist for the Erotic Awards in London. She has been featured in *The New York Times, Newsweek,* SexTV, CNN Headline News, Fox News, Spike TV, Playboy Radio, *The Village Voice,* G4TV, and Digital Village Radio. Regina lives in California with her dog, Jedi, and her horse, Rockstar.

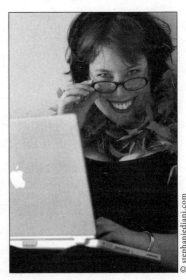

© stephaniediani.com

Acknowledgments

I cannot write in isolation, and this book would not have happened without the support of my community:

Monique, who reminded me that if we don't give gratitude for the blessings we have, there won't be room for the new blessings that are on the way.

Kelli, who wrote the online dating lessons when I was in danger of missing my final deadline.

Jenni, who encouraged and cajoled and bullied me into achieving my lifelong dream, and who helped me believe I could do it.

Janet and Yoli, who kept me on track with my day job while giving me the flexibility to keep writing.

Scott, whose belief never wavered.

Mike, who aptly described the writing process as "flying a pancake through the eye of a camel."

The experts who dropped everything and made time for me, whose names you'll find throughout the lessons.

The members of the Sex Drive Forum, who contributed their experiences and insights every step of the way, and who teach me new things every day.

And finally, lovers past and present, online and off and back again, who taught me so much of what is in these pages.

Selected Titles from Seal Press

For more than thirty years, Seal Press has published groundbreaking books.
By women. For women. Visit our website at www.sealpress.com. and our blog
at www.sealpress.com/blog.

GETTING OFF: A WOMAN'S GUIDE TO MASTURBATION by Jamye Waxman, illustrations by
Molly Crabapple. $14.94, 1-58005-219-3. Empowering and female-positive, this is a
comprehensive guide for women on the history and mechanics of the oldest and most
common sexual practice.

THE BIGGER, THE BETTER, THE TIGHTER THE SWEATER edited by Samantha Schoech and Lisa
Taggart. $14.95, 1-58005-210-X. A refreshingly honest and funny collection of essays on
how women view their bodies.

SEX AND BACON: WHY I LOVE THINGS THAT ARE VERY, VERY BAD FOR ME by Sarah Katherine
Lewis. $14.95, 1-58005-228-2. A sensual—and sometimes raunchy—book celebrating the
intersection of sex and food.

DIRTY GIRLS: EROTICA FOR WOMEN edited by Rachel Kramer Bussel. $15.95, 1-58005-
251-7. A collection of tantalizing and steamy stories compiled by prolific erotica writer
Rachel Kramer Bussel.

BETTER THAN I EVER EXPECTED: STRAIGHT TALK ABOUT SEX AFTER SIXTY by Joan Price.
$15.95, 1-58005-152-9. A warm, witty, and honest book that contends with the challenges
and celebrates the delights of older-life sexuality.

CONFESSIONS OF A NAUGHTY MOMMY: HOW I FOUND MY LOST LIBIDO by Heidi Raykeil.
$14.95, 1-58005-157-X. The Naughty Mommy shares her bedroom woes and woo-hoos
with other mamas who are rediscovering their sex lives after baby and are ready to think
about it, talk about it, and *do* it.